SAUNDERS PHYSICAL ACTIVITIES SERIES

Edited by

MARYHELEN VANNIER, Ed.D.

Professor and Director, Women's Division
Department of Health and Physical Education
Southern Methodist University

and

HOLLIS F. FAIT, Ph.D.

Professor of Physical Education
School of Physical Education
University of Connecticut

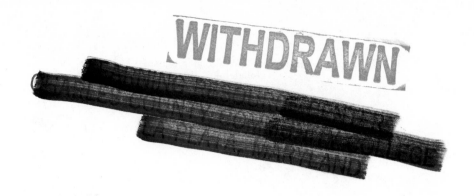

GYMNASTIC ROUTINES FOR MEN

WILLIAM VINCENT

Professor of Physical Education
San Fernando Valley State College

W. B. SAUNDERS COMPANY

PHILADELPHIA • LONDON • TORONTO

W. B. Saunders Company: West Washington Square
                          Philadelphia, Pa.   19105

                          12 Dyott Street
                          London WC1A   1DB

                          833 Oxford Street
                          Toronto 18, Ontario

Saunders Physical Activities Series

Gymnastic Routines For Men   SBN 0-7216-9045-9

Print No.   9   8   7   6   5   4   3   2   1

EDITORS' FOREWORD

Every period of history, as well as every society, has its own profile. Our own world of the last third of the twentieth century is no different. Whenever we step back to look at ourselves, we can see excellences and failings, strengths and weaknesses, that are peculiarly ours.

One of our strengths as a nation is that we are a sports-loving people. Today more persons — and not just young people — are playing, watching, listening to, and reading about sports and games. Those who enjoy themselves most are the men and women who actually *play* the game: the "doers."

You are reading this book now for either of two very good reasons. First, you want to learn — whether in a class or on your own — how to play a sport well, and you need clear, easy-to-follow instructions to develop the special skills involved. If you want to be a successful player, this book will be of much help to you.

Second, you may already have developed skill in this activity, but want to improve your performance through assessing your weaknesses and correcting your errors. You want to develop further the skills you have now and to learn and perfect additional ones. You realize that you will enjoy the activity even more if you know more about it.

In either case, this book can contribute greatly to your success. It offers "lessons" from a real professional: from an outstandingly successful coach, teacher, or performer. All the authors in the *Saunders Physical Activities Series* are experts and widely recognized in their specialized fields. Some have been members or coaches of teams of national prominence and Olympic fame.

This book, like the others in our Series, has been written to make it easy for you to help yourself to learn. The authors and the editors want you to become more self-motivated and to gain a greater understanding of, appreciation for, and proficiency in the exciting world of *movement*. All the activities described in this Series — sports, games, dance, body conditioning, and weight and figure control activities — require skillful, efficient movement. That's what physical activity is all about. Each book contains descriptions and helpful tips about the nature, value, and purpose of an activity, about the purchase and care of equipment, and about the fundamentals of each movement skill involved. These books also tell you about common errors and how to avoid making them, about ways in which you can improve your performance, and about game rules and strategy, scoring, and special techniques. Above all, they should tell you how to get the most pleasure and benefit from the time you spend.

Our purpose is to make you a successful *participant* in this age of sports activities. If you are successful, you will participate often — and this will give you countless hours of creative and recreative fun. At the same time, you will become more physically fit.

"Physical fitness" is more than just a passing fad or a slogan. It is a condition of your body which determines how effectively you can perform your daily work and play and how well you can meet unexpected demands on your strength, your physical skills, and your endurance. How fit you are depends largely on your participation in vigorous physical activity. Of course no one sports activity can provide the kind of total workout of the body required to achieve optimal fitness; but participation with vigor in any activity makes a significant contribution to this total. Consequently, the activity you will learn through reading this book can be extremely helpful to you in developing and maintaining physical fitness now and throughout the years to come.

These physiological benefits of physical activity are important beyond question. Still, the pure pleasure of participation in physical activity will probably provide your strongest motivation. The activities taught in this Series are *fun*, and they provide a most satisfying kind of recreation for your leisure hours. Also they offer you great personal satisfaction in achieving success in skillful performance — in the realization that you are able to control your body and its movement and to develop its power and beauty. Further, there can be a real sense of fulfillment in besting a skilled opponent or in exceeding a goal you have set for yourself. Even when you fall short of such triumphs, you can still find satisfaction in the effort you have made to meet a challenge. By participating in sports you can gain greater respect for yourself, for others, and for "the rules of the game." Your skills in leadership and fellowship will be sharpened and improved. Last, but hardly least, you will make new friends among others who enjoy sports activities, both as participants and as spectators.

We know you're going to enjoy this book. We hope that it — and the others in our Series — will make you a more skillful and more enthusiastic performer in all the activities you undertake.

Good luck!

Maryhelen Vannier

Hollis Fait

CONTENTS

Chapter 8

Chapter 9

Chapter 10

CHAPTER 1

INTRODUCTION AND TERMINOLOGY

Gymnastics are fun. Children love to tumble, flip, swing, jump, roll, and perform all sorts of gyrations. Even older students in the secondary schools or college find it a most enjoyable activity. You will enjoy it too, for it offers not only the chance to learn new and exciting skills, but to learn body control and grace. The ultimate objective of gymnastics is to be able to combine separate skills into a smoothly flowing, well coordinated routine of movements. The value of such an exercise is found not only in the difficulty of the individual skills but in the manner in which they are combined. How many times have you seen an expert gymnast perform obviously difficult maneuvers, but have said to yourself, "That looks so easy!" It is one of the purposes of this book to help you develop that control, grace, and elegance that is necessary to "make things look easy."

This book will lead you through a series of related skills in each of the various events and then show you how to combine them into a routine. Simple moves will be introduced first, and a basic routine will be developed; then more difficult moves will be added until you have gradually evolved into a skilled performer. But before we begin our lessons, some background material will need to be introduced.

LEARNING GYMNASTICS SKILLS

Some of you may be thinking at this point that gymnastics are not for you because you may get hurt. Gymnastics, under the direction of qualified instructors, introduced in the proper sequences of simple to complex, and utilizing some common sense safety precautions, are no more dangerous than other activities taught in the schools. Chapter 2 will discuss some of the safety aspects of the sport, but you will feel better and learn faster if you will follow some of these basic rules.

1. Start with very elementary skills. Make them so simple that you are guaranteed success on the first few trials. There is nothing so stimulating as early success. With a continuous background of positive reinforcement, your desire to learn more will grow with each lesson.

2. Progress at your own rate. Listen carefully to your teacher and take his advice, but remember that every individual progresses at a different rate. Do not attempt difficult maneuvers until you have mastered the more basic ones.

3. Follow the suggested order of learning in this book. It is designed to help you progress from simple to complex on each event.

4. Implement the basic safety rules outlined in Chapter 2.

NOMENCLATURE OF GYMNASTICS

Gymnastics, like many other sports, has a unique set of words that describe the activity. In learning the skills, discussing your progress, or describing routines, the following terms are likely to be used.

I. Naming of Positions

There are three axes to the human body: breadth, length, and depth. The breadth axis runs from side to side, the length axis runs from head to toe, and the depth axis runs from front to back. The position of the gymnast at any given time is determined by comparing the breadth axis of the body to the length axis of the apparatus. On the parallel bars, the horizontal bar, the side horse, the long horse, and the trampoline, the length axis of the apparatus is obvious. The length axis of the rings is determined by imagining a bar placed between the rings so that a person could hang from it. This bar represents the length axis of the rings. Floor exercise has no length axis since it is performed on a square mat.

When the breadth axis of the gymnast is parallel to the length axis of the apparatus, it is called a side position. Hanging from the horizontal bar with a double over or under grip is an example of a side position. On the side horse, a side position is represented by supporting your body on the pommels with the front or rear of your body against the horse.

When the broad axis of the gymnast is perpendicular to the long axis of the apparatus, it is called a cross position. Supporting yourself on the parallel bars with your legs hanging between the bars is one example. Sitting on the side horse between the pommels as if you were going to ride the horse is another example of a cross position.

If the gymnast is facing the apparatus, it is called a position frontways, and if his back is toward the apparatus, it is called a position rearways. Likewise, if the apparatus is on your left, it is a position left, and if it is on your right, it is a position right. You can readily see that there is a number of possible combinations of these positions. Standing on the ground at the end of the parallel bars with your hands on the rails, ready to jump up to a support is called a cross position frontways. Dismounting from the horizontal bar so that it is behind you results in a side position rearways. Jumping off the parallel bars to the side so that one hand is on the bar for stability results in a cross position right or left, depending upon whether the bars are on your right or left. The following diagram illustrates all of these possible positions on the side horse. Let the long line represent the broad axis of the performer (his shoulders), and the small line represent his nose (the direction in which he is facing).

The numbered positions are as follows:
1. Cross position frontways
2. Cross position rearways
3. Side position frontways
4. Side position rearways
5. Cross position left
6. Cross position right
7. Side position right
8. Side position left
9. Side position on the horse
10. Cross position on the horse

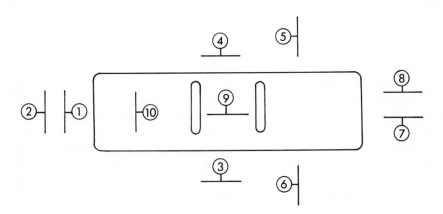

Similar diagrams could be drawn for the other pieces of apparatus. Stationary positions such as mounts, dismounts, and balances or
supports should be described by using this type of language.

II. Naming of Movements

Movements of the human body may be performed around any
one of the three axes. Movements around the breadth axis are described as being either forward or backward, or clockwise or counterclockwise. With an imaginary clock on the left shoulder of the gymnast (imagine he is looking at the clock so that the 12 is up, the 6
down, the 3 in front, and the 9 behind), the performer is considered
to be moving backwards if he moves in a counterclockwise direction,
and forward if he moves clockwise. Under these conditions, a backward flip on the trampoline would be counterclockwise, and forward flip would be clockwise. These same directions apply to somersaults, rolls, handsprings, or dives on any of the apparatus.

Movements around the length axis are called twisting moves.
They are described using the same terms that are used in marching.
With the gymnast standing on the imaginary clock, the 12 is is front,
the 6 behind, the 3 to his right, and 9 to his left. Right-hand turns or
twists are clockwise, and left-hand turns are counterclockwise. When
the gymnast is upside down, such as in a headstand or handstand,
the clock is imagined to stay on his feet and thus follows him upside
down. Jumping pirouettes and somersaults containing twisting actions are probably the most common examples of movements around
the length axis. Usually these twisting movements are in combination with another type of movement, such as a handstand or somersault.

Movements around the depth axis are also considered to be right
or left. This time, the clock is in front of the performer and facing
him. The cartwheel is the best example of this type of movement. If
you do a cartwheel to your right (right hand goes down first), you are
moving clockwise around the depth axis. If you go left (left hand
goes down first), you are moving counterclockwise. Can you think of
any other movements that are performed around the depth axis?

While we frequently use common names for many of the skills in
gymnastics, every move could be described by using the terminology
just discussed. A back flip, in the technical language, becomes a 360
degree somersault counterclockwise around the breadth axis, and a
shoulder stand on the parallel bars becomes a cross support on the
upper arms in an inverted position. For the more common skills, the
colloquial name is acceptable, but for the new moves, or for precise
communication, the technical name is preferred.

Each piece of apparatus also has some unique names and terms associated with it. As you read the various chapters, these terms will be described and defined.

OBJECTIVES OF ELEMENTARY GYMNASTICS COURSES

At the conclusion of a course in gymnastics following the procedures outlined in this book, you should be able to:
1. Demonstrate basic skills on each of the pieces of apparatus, such as kips, rolls, swings, balances, springs, and strength and flexibility moves.
2. Show improvement in upper body strength as compared to the beginning of the course. You will improve the: (a) number of chins you can perform on the horizontal bar; (b) number of dips you can perform on the parallel bars; (c) time it takes you to climb a 20 foot rope; (d) effort required to maintain your body in various holding positions on the apparatus.
3. Demonstrate your spatial awareness and orientation. Specifically, you will be able to perform somersaults and twists without losing your orientation, and be able to land in various body positions on the trampoline or the mats so as to avoid injury.
4. Describe the axes of the body and how they relate to positions and movements on the apparatus.
5. Change direction and body positions on the various pieces of apparatus with smooth flowing movements. You will exhibit gracefulness, proper body position, and continuity of motion.
6. Evaluate the performance of routines and enjoy attending and participating as a spectator in competitive gymnastics meets.

It is assumed that you are a beginner in gymnastics and you are unable to meet objectives 1, 3, 4, 5, and 6. However, in order to measure your progress on number 2, give yourself each of these tests to establish a basis for comparison at the conclusion of the course. Were you never to practice these specific tests, the activities described in this book would still cause a significant increase in your strength and you would improve in each test. Of course, you can accelerate that improvement by doing your maximum number of chins and dips three times per week and climbing the rope several times per day.

CHAPTER 2

SAFETY AND SPOTTING

A safe program of gymnastics can be evolved by the use of four general principles of safety.

1. The first principle of safety is that common sense should be used by both instructors and participants. You should never attempt any skill in gymnastics without adequate instruction, or try any difficult skill without your teacher's permission. Proper teaching progressions and leadup skills will greatly reduce the possibility of injury in moves that require you to build skill upon skill until you reach some final objective. Obviously, proper class organization is necessary, and horseplay is to be strictly prohibited. Most of the time, the responsibility to use common sense falls upon the student. Even in a well organized and directed class, you must still follow the rules established by the instructor. A student who does not follow rules and exhibits irresponsible behavior assumes the responsibility for any injury he may cause or incur.

2. Magnesium carbonate, commonly called gymnastics chalk, should be used at all times on any piece of apparatus that requires a grip with the hands, such as the rope, the side horse, the horizontal bar, the parallel bars, and the rings. Chalk absorbs perspiration and allows you to have a more secure grip on the apparatus, thus reducing the possibility of slipping.

3. Most pieces of apparatus are adaptable according to height. The apparatus should be lowered for early learning and raised for more advanced work. You should learn how to raise and lower the apparatus and secure it in place so that you may adapt it to your individual needs. Mats should be placed around and under all of the apparatus and anywhere a fall might occur. Recently, a special mat consisting of six to eight inches of foam padding has been developed. It has proven very successful in absorbing impact and may be utilized for particularly difficult landings or dismounts.

4. Skills which are particularly complicated or complex should be spotted during the early learning phase. Later on, when mastery of the skill is accomplished, as determined by the instructor or coach, further spotting may not be necessary.

Spotting in gymnastics is defined as the manipulation of the performer either by direct use of the hands or by means of a belt tied around the waist of the gymnast. The objective of spotting may be to prevent injury, to assist the gymnast in performing his skill, or both.

A safety spot in gymnastics is not primarily concerned with assisting the performer to accomplish the skill, but is designed to prevent falls. To execute a safety spot, the instructor or spotter must first determine where the fall might occur and place himself in that position. Then he must determine how he will grab or hold the performer to allow for maximum control of his body. In all spotting techniques by hand, the spotter should grab or hold the upper body of the performer whenever a spot is required. The purpose of this technique is to keep his head and shoulders off the mat, since this is the most delicate part of the body. A spotter who grabs or tackles the performer around the knees or legs is likely to cause an injury rather than prevent one.

The assistance spot is not primarily concerned with preventing falls or injury, and may even be executed on beginning moves. This spot is designed to assist in accomplishing the skill. To perform this spot adequately, you must know the desired action of the performer; then determine how you should put your hands on his body to assist him to complete the skill.

Good spotting technique is not easily learned. It requires a great deal of practice and an understanding of gymnastics moves, but being a good gymnast does not necessarily make one a good spotter. When spotting by hand, certain techniques are most helpful. The first one is to stand close to the performer. Regardless of the hand placement on the performer, you cannot properly assist or hold the gymnast up if you are more than half an armlength away. Many times, the entire arms and body of the spotter are in direct contact with the gymnast. A second technique is to be in the right place at the right time; anticipate the fall and be there before it happens.

Paying close attention to the task is another technique of extreme importance. Many times, classmates will be looking around the gymnasium or paying attention to some other activity when their performer is ready to attempt a move. Letting your mind wander is sometimes a costly error. Finally, always follow the rule: "When in doubt, spot!" The consequences of not spotting when it is indicated are much more serious than those of spotting when it may not have been necessary.

Spotting belts are most helpful in teaching gymnastics. These pieces of equipment usually consist of a large belt with ropes attached, strapped around the performer's waist so that a spotter on either side of the performer can hold the rope. On a hand belt, the ropes are about four feet long on each side and the spotters stand next to the performer to hold the ropes. On an overhead belt, the ropes run up to the ceiling and through a series of pulleys so that a

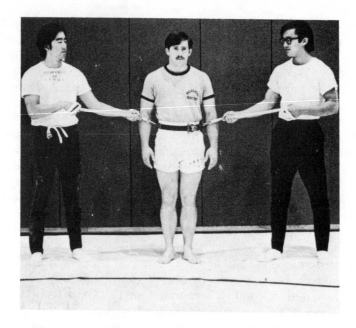

single spotter can stand to the side of the performer and actually lift him into the air.

Some belts are designed to allow rotation around the length axis as well as the breadth axis of the body. These are called twisting belts. The spotting belt should be tightened around the waist to a point where it will not slide up and down the body, but should not be so tight that it is uncomfortable to the performer.

When using a hand belt, the spotter should hold the end of the rope in one hand to allow the performer sufficient slack to make his preliminary moves. Then, when the critical part of the skill is attempted, the other hand should slide up the rope and right next to the belt, so that maximum control can be maintained.

To use the overhead spotting belt with the pulley system on the ceiling, allow some slack for the preliminary moves of the skill, but pull the rope taut when the critical part of the skill is attempted. You must know what preliminary moves are going to be attempted and when the critical part of the skill will occur. Then you must take the slack out of the rope in such a way that the gymnast is not jerked or pulled prematurely. One of the most common errors in spotting with the overhead belt is to leave the ropes too loose. Since it takes time to pull the slack out, either the performer is jerked or the spot comes too late. Conversely, too much slack may cause the performer to be tangled in the ropes. Practice and experience will dictate the proper amount of slack. If you are willing to take time to determine the proper position of the ropes, almost any skill can be spotted by an overhead belt.

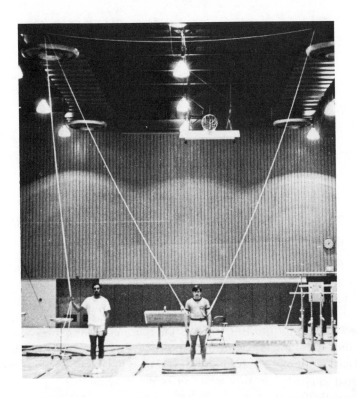

The parallel bars present a unique problem in spotting. You must be careful not to place your arms over the top of the bars, since the performer could come down and pin your arms across the bar and perhaps cause injury to you. For hand spots on the parallel bars, stay close and catch the performer if and when he falls below the level of the bars. Most gymnasts will be able to break their own falls by grabbing the bar, but the spotter can assist by keeping the performer's head and shoulders off the ground.

When spotting tumbling or floor exercise, it is most important that you anticipate the place on the floor where the skill to be spotted will occur. Sometimes it is necessary to run along with the performer and spot him several times during a tumbling pass. Single moves in early learning stages, such as back handsprings, may be more easily spotted while you are kneeling; you can sometimes get underneath the performer more easily than you could while standing.

Gymnastics is a most enjoyable activity. It offers some unique experiences that cannot be gained in other sports. With correct spotting techniques, common sense, and proper safety precautions, this activity can be a most valuable part of your physical education experience.

CHAPTER 3

TUMBLING AND FLOOR EXERCISE

In the past, tumbling and floor exercise were considered to be two separate events. Modern thinking, however, has combined the two into one composite event in which tumbling is the major element, with leaps, balances, and flexibility and strength parts interspersed between tumbling passes. This "new" floor exercise event is more dramatic and pleasing to the observer because it requires the performer to demonstrate many different types of skills. This chapter will assist you in learning some of these movements.

Most secondary school students have been introduced to basic tumbling skills such as forward and backward rolls. Let's start with a quick review of these two and then proceed into some more difficult maneuvers.

A good teacher will not ask his students to perform skills for which they are not properly prepared. You may be of the opinion that a forward roll is probably the easiest skill in tumbling; however, some prior conditioning may be required to assure flexibility of the spine and neck. So before attempting this skill, do some stretching exercises and loosening movements for the neck muscles. Then, perhaps some warmups on log rolls would help you become accustomed to rolling and turning over. To perform a log roll, simply lie down on a mat and roll sideways several times. This log roll can be modified to a race across the mats, or a relay between squads. All of these activities can help prepare you both mentally and physically for the coming skills.

FORWARD ROLL

The forward roll may be performed from several starting positions, but the easiest to learn is from the squat position. Squat down

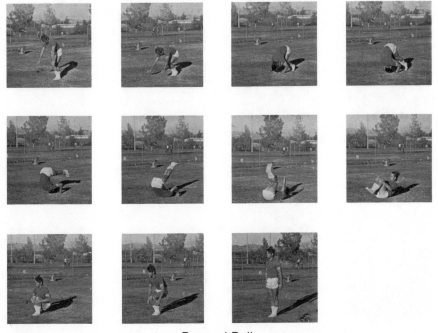

Forward Roll.

on the mat and place your hands shoulder width apart on the mat in front of you. Now raise your hips over your head and place the back of your neck on the mat. Kick with your feet to push yourself over. On the next try, keep your knees together and bent as you roll, and finally grab your shins halfway through the roll and pull yourself up to a stand. A little speed will help you stand up more easily.

BACKWARD ROLL

The steps in performing the backward roll are the same as for the forward roll but are taken in the reverse order. First, squat down and grab your shin bones, and form a tight ball with your body. Then roll backwards until the back of your neck is on the mat. As you approach this position, place your hands on the mat next to your head with your palms down and your thumbs pointing toward your ears. Now push hard with your hands and place your feet on the ground. Remember to keep tucked up in a tight ball and roll fast enough to develop the momentum needed to carry your body up and over your hands and head. If you find yourself stuck upside down in the middle of the skill, you are probably not rolling fast enough or you are not staying tucked up. Also remember that your hands not

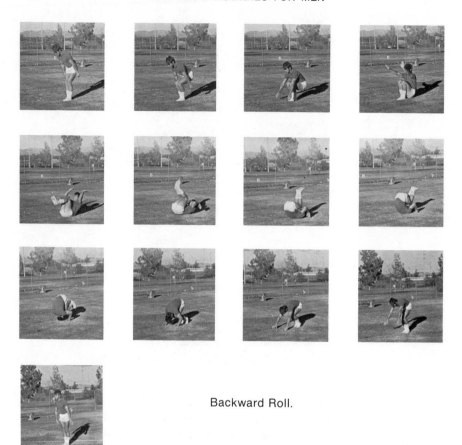

Backward Roll.

only push you over, but help support your body so that your total
weight does not rest on your head and neck. Placement of the hands
is probably the most critical part of this skill. Spotters may help by
lifting your hips up and over your head and removing some of the
weight as you pass over the top.

STRADDLE LEAP

Here is a move that is both a leap and a flexibility skill. Before
you try this one, touch your toes a few times and stretch out the
muscles on the insides of your legs. To perform this leap properly,
jump into the air and touch your toes with your hands while your
legs are spread apart and parallel to the mat. Try not to reach down
with your hands, but lift your legs up to meet them. Obviously, the
higher you jump and the farther you spread your legs, the more
effective is the leap.

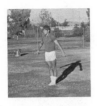
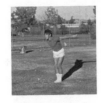
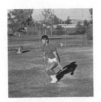
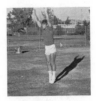

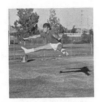
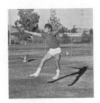
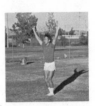

Straddle Leap.

SQUAT BALANCE

This skill is one of the most elementary balance moves. With your feet about one foot apart, squat down and spread your knees apart. Now place your hands on the mat between your knees, with your fingers spread wide apart. In this position, your elbows should come in contact with the insides of your knees. Press out with your elbows and in with your knees to stabilize yourself. Now lean forward until your head almost touches the mat and your feet come off the mat about one inch. In this position, you will somewhat resemble a frog; in fact, this balance is sometimes called a "frog stand".

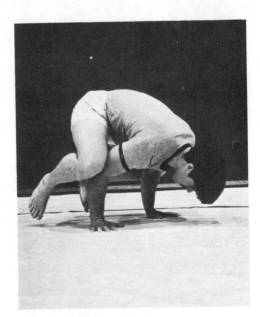

Squat Balance.

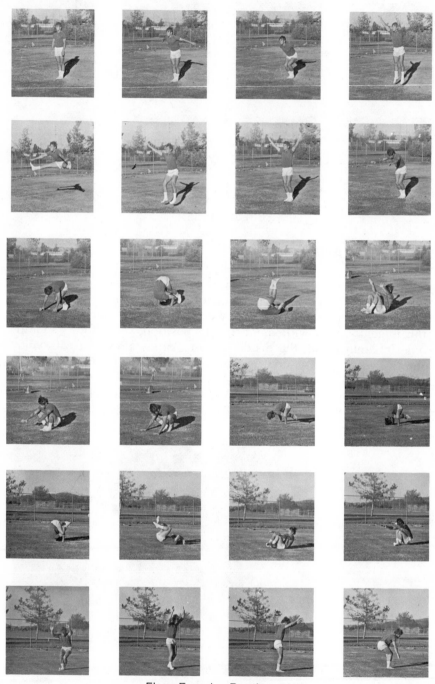

Floor Exercise Routine #1.

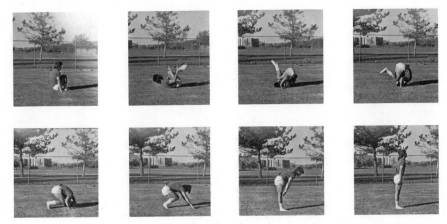

Figure Continued.

ROUTINE #1

Remembering that our philosophy in this book is to combine simple moves into routines, let's use the four skills we have learned in floor exercise to make up our first routine. Arrange a row of mats, or stand in one corner of a 40' by 40' floor exercise pad, and try the following combination:

1. Straddle jump.
2. Forward roll and finish in a squat position.
3. Place hands down and lean forward to a squat balance (hold for 3 seconds).
4. Place your head on the mat and roll forward again, but as you go over the top, cross your legs.
5. Stand up with crossed legs and turn around by uncrossing your legs.
6. Squat and roll backwards to a standing position.

You can probably do all of these skills individually, but remember that a routine must be smooth and flowing so that each skill blends with the next. Strive for this in your practice so that the entire exercise becomes one well coordinated movement. When this is accomplished, you are ready to move to more difficult skills.

LEG CIRCLES

Here is a challenging skill that requires flexibility, balance, and coordination of the arms and legs. Once again, assume the squat position with your hands on the mat in front of you, but this time place your right leg to the side with the knee straight, so that you are

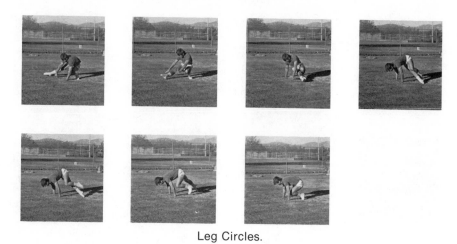

Leg Circles.

now squatting on just your left leg. Swing your right leg around in front and lean back on your left leg so that the swinging leg passes under both of your hands. Quickly replace your hands on the mat and shift your body weight from your left leg to both hands. Your right leg should now be under your body and extended toward your left side. Lean hard on your hands and continue the circle with your right leg. Lift your left foot up so that the leg can pass under it and once again shift the weight back to your left foot. This should bring you back to the original position. Notice that your right leg must pass alternately under your hands and your left leg. Shifting your weight from hands to leg is critical, since you must alternately balance on each of them. Also, be sure to keep your right knee straight, especially as it passes under your left leg. Of course, this entire maneuver could be reversed so that your right leg goes in the other direction, or so that you use your left leg as the "rope" to jump over.

STRADDLE FORWARD ROLL

This is one of several possible variations on the forward roll. It begins in the same manner as the forward roll, but as your legs come down, they are spread wide apart with your knees straight. Your hands should be placed on the mat between your legs. From this position, keep your momentum going by keeping your head down, leaning forward and pushing hard on the mat with your hands. Do not stand up and extend your hips until you have reached an upright position with your upper body parallel to the mat. Of course, the wider you spread your legs, the easier it will be to stand up. This is where the flexibility part comes in. You will have a tendency to bend

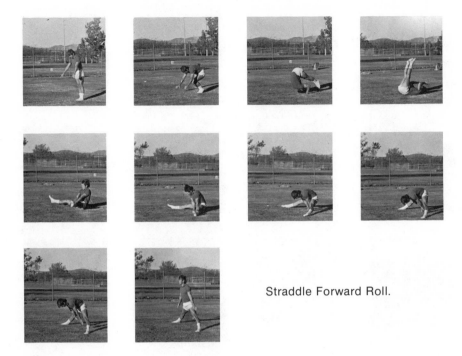

Straddle Forward Roll.

your knees at first, but this skill must be performed with straight legs.

CARTWHEEL

Cartwheels are among the most popular gymnastics skills, yet seldom are they performed properly by beginners. Since a cartwheel contains a momentary handstand, you will have to learn this first. Get down on the mat as if you were about to start a race with both hands on the mat and your right foot farther back than your left. Now kick the right foot up in the air and follow it with the left, so that you attain a momentary handstand. Do not attempt to hold this position, but be sure that you get all the way up with both feet almost above your head. After you feel comfortable with this, do it again, but switch your feet in the air so that you kick up with your right foot, and your right foot is also the first one to come down. Keep your knees straight when you do this. Now stand up with your right leg behind your left and do the same thing, but begin with your hands over your head in a standing position, throw them down at the mat and kick to a handstand position, switch legs and come down. Practice this until you become proficient. Next, draw two circles with

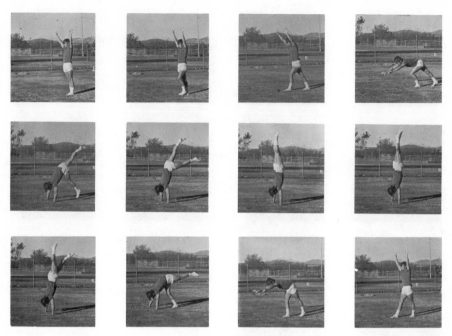

Kick to a Handstand.

chalk where your hands will touch the mat and two arrows, one entering the hand position at 45 degrees and another leaving the hand position at 45 degrees. Now stand with your left foot on the entry line and your right foot behind it, and kick to a handstand. Then come down with your right foot on the exit line and return to a standing position. This is a cartwheel at 45 degrees. After mastering this part, move your entry and exit lines closer to a straight line so that eventually your cartwheel begins and ends completely sideways. Remember that a good cartwheel begins and ends sideways and contains a momentary handstand in the middle.

(*Text continued on page 22.*)

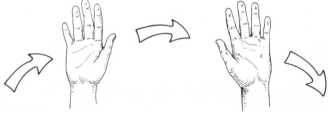

Placement of Hands for Cartwheel (as would be seen from below).

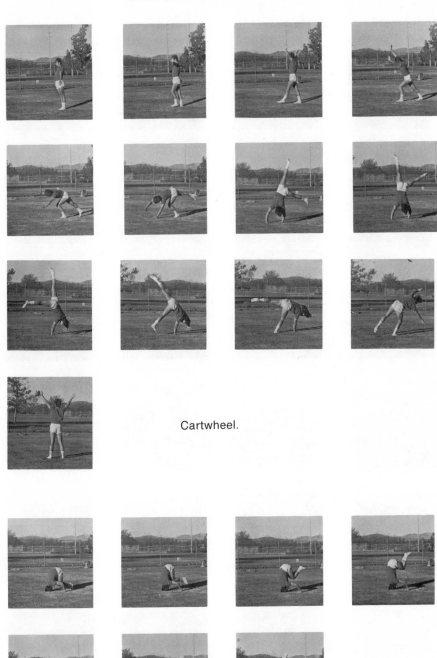

Cartwheel.

Head Stand.

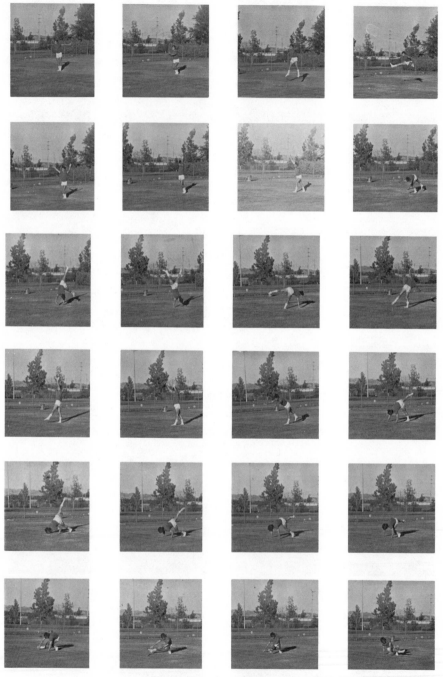

Floor Exercise Routine #2.

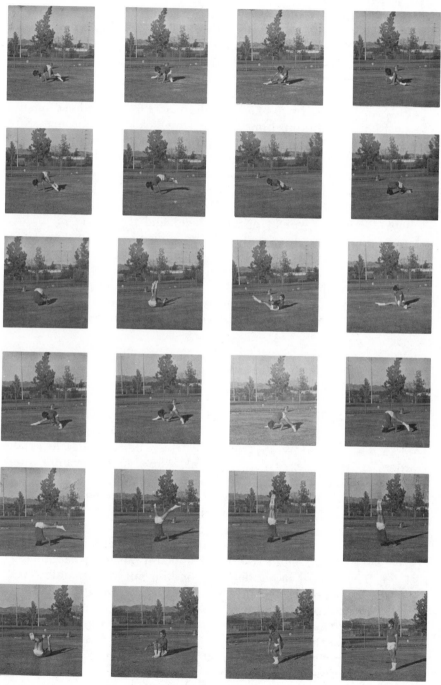

Figure Continued.

HEAD STAND

Probably sometime in your life you have tried to stand on your head. Even without instruction it is not too difficult, but by following some basic rules you should be able to learn it quickly. In all balance moves, the wider the base of support, the more stable the position. To make your head stand base as wide as possible, form a triangle with your head and two hands on the mat. Place your head in such a position that the top front part of your head is on the mat. Now walk your feet towards your head until your hips are directly over your base of support. From this position you should be able to raise your legs off of the mat and balance in an upside down squat. After you feel this balance position, slowly raise your feet until they are above your head and your body is extended into a slight arch. (Keep about 2/3 of the weight on your head and the other 1/3 divided between your two hands.) It is more difficult to keep your knees straight as you extend into the head stand. Stand up with your feet about three or four feet apart and bend at the waist until you can form the triangle on the mat. Now lean forward and push with your hands until your feet come off the mat. Slowly raise your straight legs up and together until the head stand position is accomplished.

ROUTINE #2

When you have mastered your new skills of leg circles, straddle roll, cartwheel and head stand, you are ready to incorporate them into a new routine. While these skills could be combined in various orders, try this order first and then make up your own combinations.
1. Straddle jump.
2. Cartwheel, and fall forward with both hands on the mat and your right leg raised high in the air.
3. Hop on left leg up to a squat position and circle your right leg twice around in leg circles. After the second circle, return both feet behind you into a standard pushup position.
4. Tuck your head under and straddle roll to a straddle stand.
5. Lean forward and press with straight knees to a head stand (hold 3 seconds).
6. Tuck your knees and head and roll up to a standing position.
   Remember that, whether in this combination or some other, the actions of your arms and legs should be coordinated with the skills so that your entire body action flows from one move to another.

HEAD SPRING

The head spring is a member of the kip family, for it requires the same action (as would a kip on any other apparatus) of vigorous rapid extension of the hip joint to raise the center of gravity of the body. It is this hard whip of the legs and concomitant push of the hands that will snap you up to your feet. Begin by forming a headstand triangle with your hips directly over your head and your legs straight and together behind you. Now let your hips roll forward past your head, and as you begin to feel off balance forward, whip your legs over and onto the mat. At the same time, push hard on the mat with your hands. Keep your knees straight during the whip, and bend them only as a preparation for landing.

It is important that you do not kick too soon. If you find yourself kicking straight up instead of out in front, then wait a little longer until your hips are past your base of support. On the other hand, if you wait too long your kick will be too flat and you will not be able to get your feet under you for landing. The proper timing of the kick is the most critical factor in learning the head spring. Spotters may assist by lifting your shoulders as you kick.

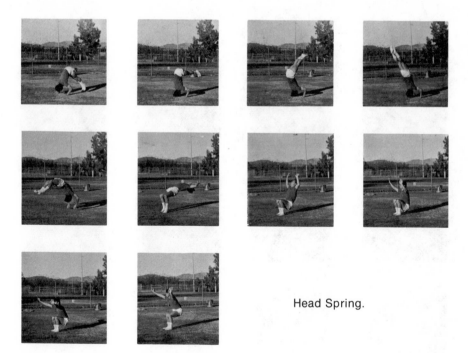

Head Spring.

FRONT HAND SPRING

Begin to learn this move by kicking to a hand stand and rolling forward out of it. Then try it from a standing position with one step. Stand with your hands above your head and raise your left foot in front of your body. Now step hard on your left foot, place your hands on the mat, and kick with your right foot up to a hand stand, immediately rolling forward to a stand. Be sure to attain the hand stand position momentarily before your roll.

Next, begin with a little run and practice the step-hop-step. As you are running (really just a fast walk), step on your right foot, then raise your hands above your head and hop on your right with your left foot in front of your body. Now step on your left foot and kick to a hand stand with your right foot. Again roll out.

When you feel competent with the step-hop-step, increase your approach speed and kick extra hard with your right foot. Snap both feet together in the air and land in the same manner as in the head spring. Do not snap your head forward until after your feet have gone over your head. Remember, a good step-hop-step approach, speed in the kick of the leg, and bringing your feet together and down as in the head spring are the key factors in completing this hand spring.

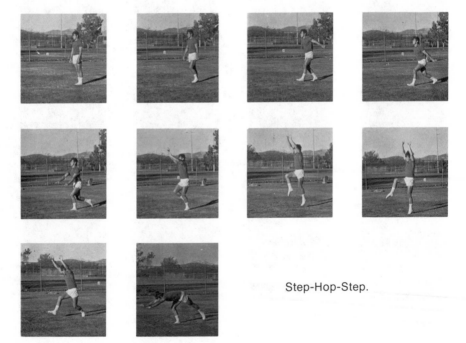

Step-Hop-Step.

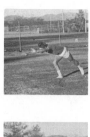 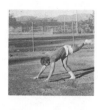 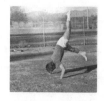

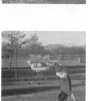 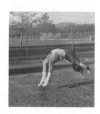 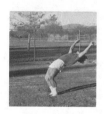 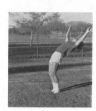

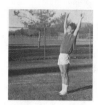

Forward Hand Spring.

Spotters may kneel on the mat where your hands will touch and lift your shoulders up when you kick, as in the head spring.

BACK HAND SPRING

This skill represents the stepping-off point for many more advance tumbling skills. This is a move that should not be attempted without personal instruction. Be sure to consult your teacher for help before attempting this move. Spotters or a hand spotting belt are usually necessary for some time before the back hand spring is attempted alone.

With your spotter kneeling at the side and behind you, practice sitting backwards as if you are sitting into a chair. Keep your back straight and perpendicular to the mat, then bend your knees to 90 degrees so that your thighs are parallel to the mat. The spotter will have to catch you when you assume this position because without him you would fall backwards. During the sit, drop your arms down and back in preparation for throwing them up and over your head. After you have learned the sit, have two spotters stand behind you and grasp each other's right wrist behind your back. Then lean backwards over their arms, looking back for the mat in a backbend

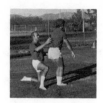 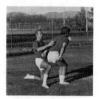

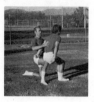

Sit for Back Hand Spring with Spotter.

position. When your hands come in contact with the mat, the spotters should lift your legs up over your head until you are in a hand stand. When your weight is on your hands, snap your feet down to the mat and push hard with your hands and return to a stand. This is called a back bend hand spring. It is performed much more slowly than a

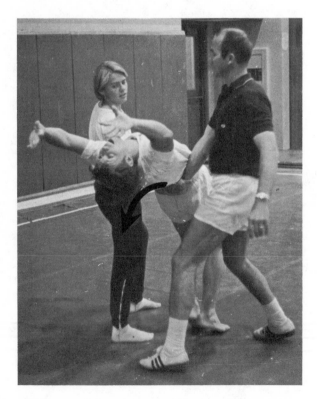

Back Bend Hand
Spring with Spotters.

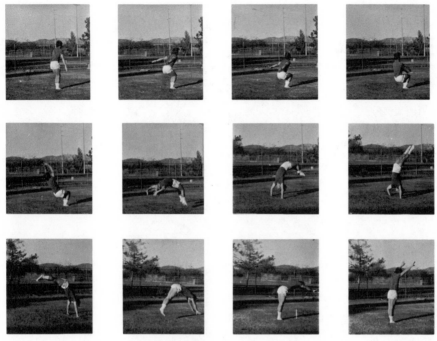

Backward Hand Spring.

regular hand spring, but allows you to experience the feeling of bending backwards to a hand stand. Practice it until you can do it with a minimum spot.

With two good spotters assisting you, you are now ready to try the complete back hand spring. Spotters may either use the double wrist grip, or kneel by your side and support your lower back with their hands. Begin with the sit back and arm swing, and then throw your arms and head backwards and jump hard from the mat. Look for the mat behind you, and place your hands on it in a hand stand position. Think to yourself "Jump backwards to a hand stand," while keeping your elbows straight. Many attempts will be necessary to master this skill. Do not be discouraged if you do not learn it on the first day.

ROUTINE #3

This routine represents a respectable combination of tumbling and floor exercise skills. If you can perform it, you may consider yourself an intermediate floor exercise performer.

1. From a standing position, perform a back hand spring and land on your right foot.

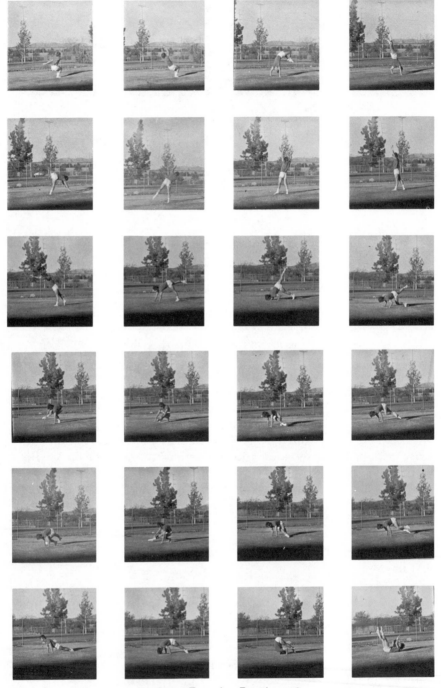

Floor Exercise Routine #3.

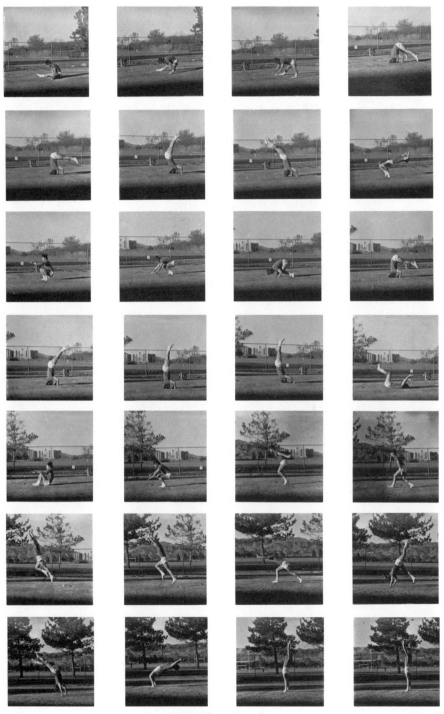

Figure Continued.

2. Turn 180 degrees and place your left foot on the mat, fall forward, and place your hands on the mat with your right foot held high in the air.

3. Hop your left leg up to a squat position and circle your right leg twice around in leg circles, returning to a pushup position.

4. Tuck your head under to a straddle roll and again place your hands on the mat in front of you.

5. Bring your legs together and do a head spring forward to a squat stand.

6. Bend forward, form a triangle, and press to a head stand (hold for 3 seconds).

7. Roll forward to a stand, take three steps and perform a front hand spring to the standing position.

You will have to practice this routine many times to develop the smooth flowing action desired. There should be no stops except in the head stand, and each move should combine into the next without jerky movements. Try to think of other combinations of the skills you have learned and make up your own routines. Have your teacher watch for continuity and smoothness while you try to "make it look easy."

CHAPTER 4

PARALLEL BARS

Almost every student has some familiarity with the parallel bars, for it is probably the most common piece of apparatus in the gymnasium. Parallel bars are normally used for performing dips, stiff arm hand walks, and simple dismounts, with little emphasis on continuity of movement from one skill to another. This chapter will help you master some of the basic skills and then put them together into several routines of increasing difficulty. Such routines more closely resemble the proper concept of gymnastics, that is, the performance of a series of exercises in a smooth, well coordinated, flowing sequence demonstrating both physical ability and artistic value.

Beginners performing on parallel bars usually find it more comfortable to have the bars adjusted fairly close together. Later, for more advanced skills, a wider adjustment may be desired, but as a start, the width of the bars should correspond to the distance between your elbow and the second knuckle of your middle finger. This allows your hips to swing freely, but still provides a straight up and down position for your arms. Set the bars high enough to allow the feet to reach the mat easily when performing an upper arm hang.

Before attempting any of the skills suggested later in this chap-

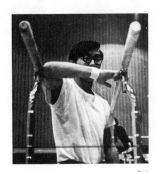

Parallel Bar Adjustment.

ter, you should practice swinging between the bars in a cross support position (see first picture below). This basic swing should be similar to the pendulum of a clock and should originate from your shoulders, not from your hips. As your legs swing forward, your arms and shoulders will naturally lean back, and as your legs and body swing backward, your arms will lean forward. This helps balance your body during the swing. A smooth, relaxed swing, with your feet rising at least as high as the bars on both ends of the swing, is the desired action. After you feel comfortable with this basic swing, you should begin work on the several skills that will later be integrated into the routines. Following is a list of these skills in a suggested learning order.

STRADDLE TRAVEL

This is an easy method of traveling along the bar, and is initiated from a cross support by straddling your legs over the bars in front of your body. Then release your hands and regrasp in front of your legs, after which your legs come together above the bars without bending at the knees to continue their forward swing. This action may be performed in a continuous action along the length of the bars.

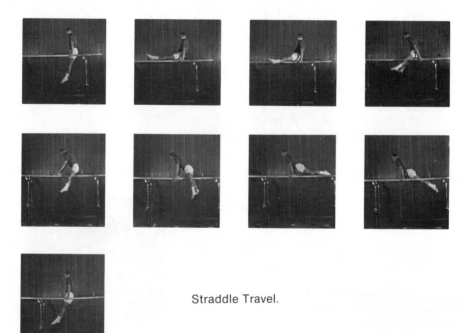

Straddle Travel.

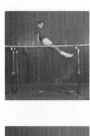 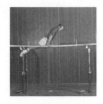 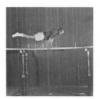

 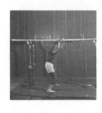

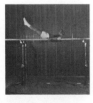 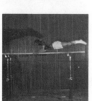

Front Dismount.

FRONT DISMOUNT

From a cross support position, while performing the basic swing, lift your legs up and over the right bar on one of the rear swings. As your legs swing over the bar, release with your left hand and regrasp the right bar; then release with your right hand as you land on the mat. Your left hand remains on the right bar for support and stability during landing. The skill could of course be performed in the opposite direction.

REAR SWING RISE

From a cross support position, while hanging by your upper arms and grasping the bars a comfortable distance in front of your

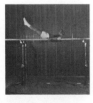 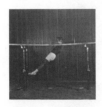 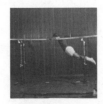 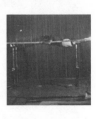

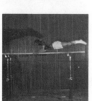 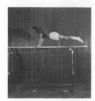 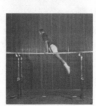

Rear Uprise.

shoulders (elbows bent at about 90 degrees), begin a pendulum swing. On one of the rear swings, shift your weight forward over your hands and off your upper arms, while simultaneously executing a pushup to a straight arm cross support. The swing is then continued forward in a straight arm position. When executing this skill, you may have a tendency to shift your hands backward rather than shifting your body weight forward and over your hands. Hand shifts should be discouraged since they are not as fluent in their motion and they usually result in a still upper position with no swing. At first your uprise will be quick and jerky, but as your pendulum swing increases in amplitude, this additional momentum may be used to make the pushup smooth and controlled.

SHOULDER OR UPPER ARM STAND

This is a balance move similar to a head stand. Since the upper arm stand contains four points of support (both hands and both arms), it is easier to perform than the head stand on the mats, which has only three points of support. From a straight arm cross support, hook your toes and knees over the bars in the rear and, without releasing

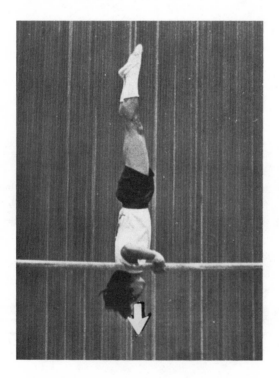

Upper Arm Stand.

your grip, lower your upper arms to the bars. Your arms should contact the bars about twelve inches in front of your hands, while your hands grasp the bars from the outside with thumbs on top and fingers underneath. From this position, walk your feet forward, raising the hips directly over the base of support formed by your two hands and two arms. Once this is accomplished, your legs and feet can be raised overhead and straightened out. Your back should maintain a slight arch while your eyes are focused on the mat below. Spotters should keep their arms *under* the bars and on the lower back of the performer.

FORWARD ROLL FROM UPPER ARM STAND

You may come down from the arm stand in exacty the opposite manner in which you got up, but you should also learn to roll forward to an upper arm hang. The roll is started by bending your hips, and then tucking your head to your chest. Your hands then release the bar and quickly regrasp in front of your arms. Care should be taken to move your arms around the side during the regrasp, and not

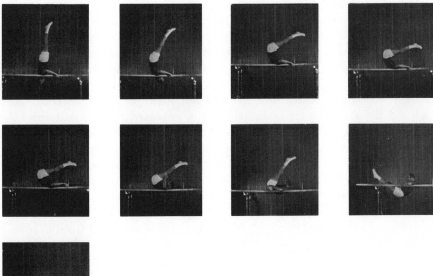

Forward Roll from Upper Arm Stand.

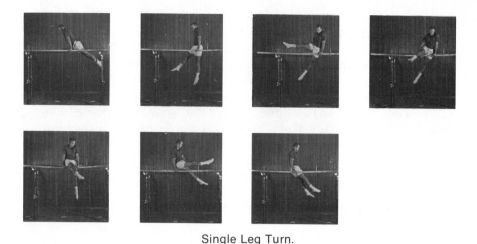

Single Leg Turn.

through a vertical plane. This will eliminate the possibility of slipping through the bars. Once you have regrasped the bar, continue your backward swing in preparation for the rear uprise. Spotters should place one arm *under* the bar and on the performer's lower back, while the other arm grasps the performer's wrist and guides his hand during the regrasp.

SINGLE LEG TURN

This skill provides a simple method of turning around between the bars and allows you to continue your routine in the opposite direction. Again from the straight arm cross support swing, lift your right leg over the left bar on one of the forward swings, placing your hips over the bar as close to your left hand as possible. Your right hand then releases the right bar and regrasps the left bar directly behind your body. You have now completed a 180 degree turn and are sitting in a straddle position on the left bar. From this position, move your left hand to the right bar and swing your right leg over the left bar into the middle. Your legs should come together in front of your body and continue backward in a smooth swing. With practice, this skill can be performed in a smooth continuous action without sitting on the bar. It may also be executed in reverse, turning around the other bar.

ROUTINE #1

After these skills have been mastered, they may be put together in the following order to constitute a smooth flowing routine:

1. From a cross stand frontward, jump to cross support.
2. Straddle travel to the center of the bars.
3. Place feet on bars behind body and press to shoulder stand (hold for 3 seconds).
4. Roll forward to upper arm hang.
5. Rear uprise to cross support.
6. Single leg turn.
7. Front dismount to cross stand on either side of the bar.

FORWARD SWING RISE

The forward swing rise, or front uprise, is the next logical skill to learn and incorporate into your routine. This skill is just the opposite of the rear uprise we learned earlier. It begins in the same manner— from an upper arm hang with a pendulum swing. However, this time the rise comes on the forward or front swing. Remember that your arms should be bent at about 90 degrees with your hands grasping the bars in front of your body. As your legs swing forward, pull your shoulders forward and up over your hands to an upper arm support. Keep your hips relatively straight throughout the swing and during the rise. It is a common error to bend the hips too much and thus make it more difficult to raise your center of gravity up and over your hands. This skill is considerably more difficult than the rear uprise, and you will probably have to practice more in order to master it. After completing the rise, your feet and legs should be in front of you and ready to swing backwards to complete the upper arm swing with straight arms.

SWING TO UPPER ARM STAND

After you have mastered the upper arm stand by kneeling on the bars and walking your feet up to the extended position, you are ready to learn another method of performing this skill which is smoother and more flowing. From a straight arm cross swinging support, as your legs rise up in the back, bend your elbows and lower your arms to the bars. Your upper arms should contact the bars in the same position as before (about one foot in front of your hands), and your head should remain in line with your body and not tucked under too much. As your legs continue to rise in the back, arch your body slightly to bring your feet right over your base of support. Keep your eyes on the mat below and balance in an upper arm stand. Caution should be taken to move your elbows sideways as your arms come in contact with the bars. This action will eliminate the possibility of

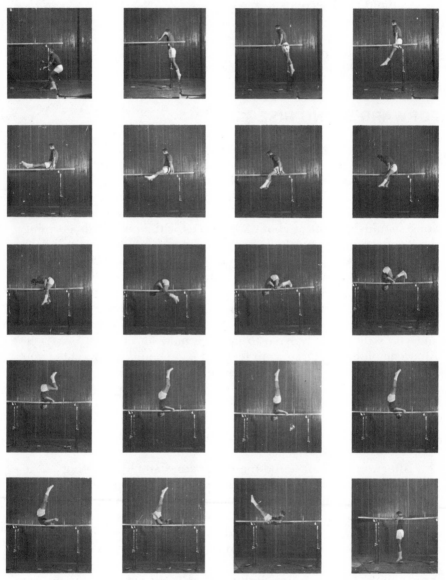

Parallel Bar Routine #1.

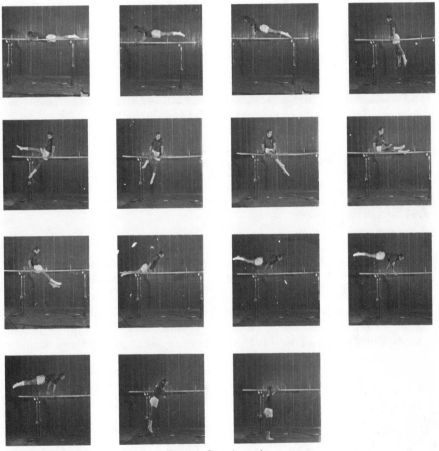

Figure Continued.

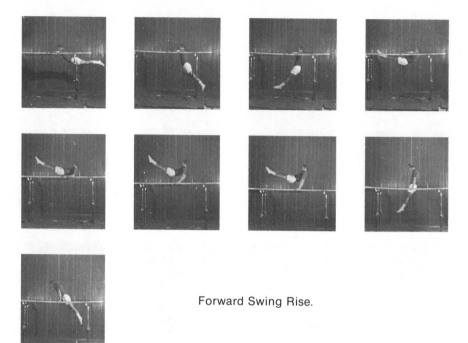

Forward Swing Rise.

falling through the bars. As your arms contact the bars, shift your weight forward so that most of it is on your arms and just a little remains on your hands. The hands are there for balance, and are not intended to carry the weight of your body. Placing the weight on your arms will also give you a more stable feeling and allow you to move your elbows sideways. Spotters may spot in the same manner

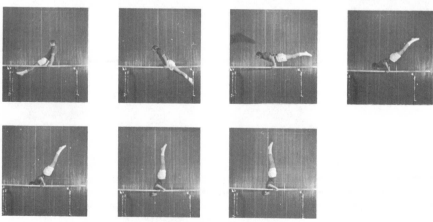

Swing to Upper Arm Stand.

described earlier, but must be ready to catch the lower back from under the bar with one arm, and the elbow with the other arm, to make sure the elbow moves sideways.

ROUTINE #2

These two new skills may now be incorporated into the first routine to increase both its difficulty and its artistic value. The routine is now as follows:
1. From a cross stand frontways, jump to a cross support on the upper arms.
2. Swing forward to a front uprise.
3. Swing the legs backward and lower to an upper arm stand (hold 3 seconds).
4. Roll forward (clockwise) to an upper arm hang and. . .
5. Rear uprise to cross support.
6. Swing legs forward to single leg turn and. . .
7. Front dismount to cross stand on either side of the bar.

UPPER ARM KIP

A kip is a vigorous and rapid extension of the hip joint for the purpose of developing momentum to raise the center of gravity of the body. It may be performed on all the events in gymnastics in one form or another. Probably one of the easiest kips to learn is the upper arm kip on the parallel bars. After completing Rountine #2, you should have no trouble learning a kip. Begin from an upper arm hang with a pendulum swing, and as your legs rise up in front, flex your hips so that your knees come almost in front of your nose and your hips are above the bar. Keep your knees straight. From this position, give a vigorous and rapid extension of your hip joint so that your legs kick out and away from you at about 45 degrees. This kick will cause your upper body to lift up and off the bars. Assist this lift by pushing down with your arms. You should finish in a cross support position with straight arms. Let your legs continue their swing backwards to complete the action. (See page 44.)

Spotters should stand on the side and reach under the bar with both arms to support the back of the leg and the middle back of the performer. As he kicks, lift with both hands; then shift the hand from his legs to the front of his chest to eliminate a forward fall which could result from too much kick and lift. This usually does not happen on the first few tries, but later the performer may kick with more force than is needed to lift his body off the bars.

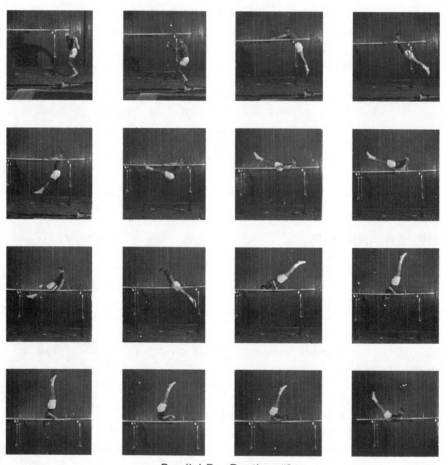

Parallel Bar Routine #2.

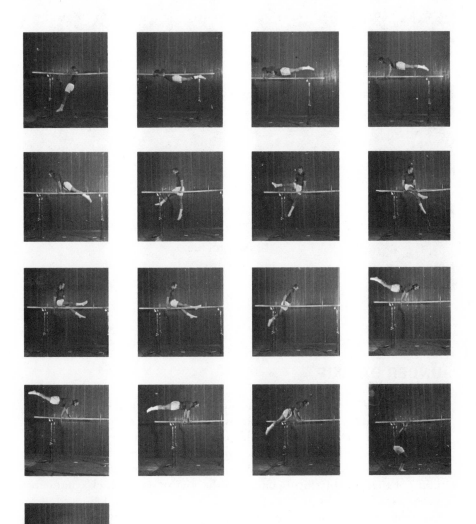

Figure Continued.

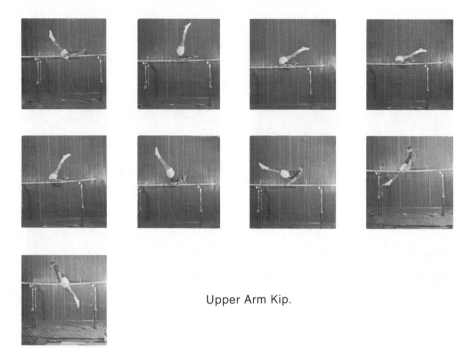

Upper Arm Kip.

UNDER BAR KIP

The kip may also be performed from under the bar. From a piked or bent body inverted hang with swing, execute the same extension of the hip joint as the end of your backward swing approaches. In this case, the kick must be harder since the center of gravity of your body must be raised from a lower position. Timing is more critical in this kip because of the swing. If the kick comes too soon or too late, the momentum from the kick will not be added to the momentum from the swing, and the support position cannot be attained. Begin your kick as you pass the center of the swing and extend it fully at the back of the swing.

FRONT DISMOUNT WITH ONE HALF TURN

To increase the difficulty of the front dismount, add a one half twist. The twist may be performed in either direction, but the most

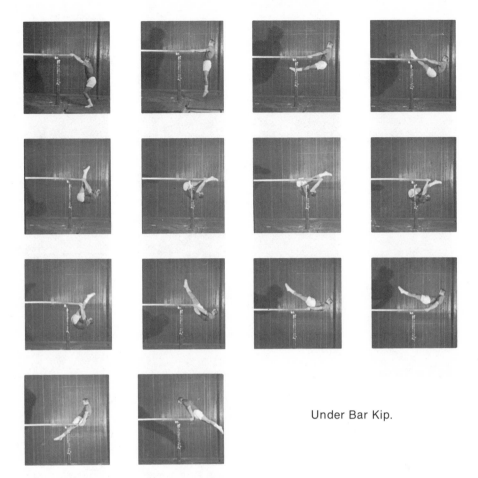

Under Bar Kip.

effective and impressive turn is away from the bar. On a front dismount over the left bar, the outward turn would be in a counterclockwise direction around the long axis of the body. Quick hand changes are required to execute this skill properly. It begins in the same manner as the normal front dismount, over the left bar, with the right hand releasing and regrasping the left bar; but as you release your left hand, you must begin a counterclockwise turn. During the turn, your left hand should reach around behind your body and again regrasp the left bar to stabilize your landing. Of course, your right hand must also release the left bar so that the turn can be completed. Begin learning this skill with the bars at a low level so that the hand changes can be practiced in slow motion. Then raise the bars as you become more competent.

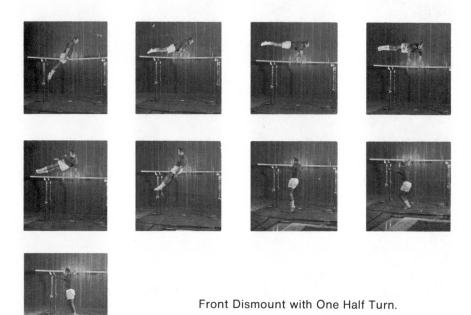

Front Dismount with One Half Turn.

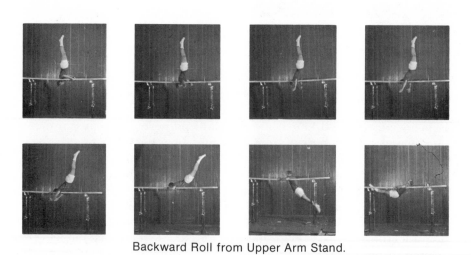

Backward Roll from Upper Arm Stand.

BACKWARD ROLL FROM UPPER ARM STAND

You have already learned to roll forward from the upper arm stand, but to add variety to your routines you should also be able to roll the other way. From your upper arm stand position, tilt your head back and begin to lower your body while keeping a slight arched position. Release your grip with both hands and move them below bar level and around the side, and regrasp in front of your shoulders. This regrasp should be made as quickly as possible to increase stability and eliminate any slipping on your upper arms. After your body comes down and between the bars, let your legs swing forward to produce a continuity of action.

ROUTINE #3

With the completion of the kip and the dismount with one half twist, you are ready to incorporate them into the routines you have already learned. Here is a description of your final routine on the parallel bars:

1. From a cross stand frontways, jump to a cross support on the upper arms.
2. Swing forward to a front uprise.
3. Swing the legs backward and lower to an upper arm position (do not hold).
4. Immediately roll forward (clockwise) to an upper arm hang, and. . .
5. Rear uprise to cross support.
6. Swing legs forward to a single leg turn and. . .
7. Swing the legs backward and again lower to an upper arm stand (hold for 3 seconds).
8. Roll backwards (counterclockwise) and swing the legs up in front and above the bar to an upper arm kip position.
9. Kip to a cross support with straight arms and swing the legs backwards, and. . .
10. Swing your legs up and over the right bar to a front dismount right with one half turn clockwise to a cross stand right.

When performed properly, this routine represents an intermediate level of achievement on the parallel bars. Care should be taken to keep your legs straight, your toes pointed, and your body in proper alignment during the entire exercise. Strive for excellence of execution after you have mastered the individual skills, and "make it look easy."

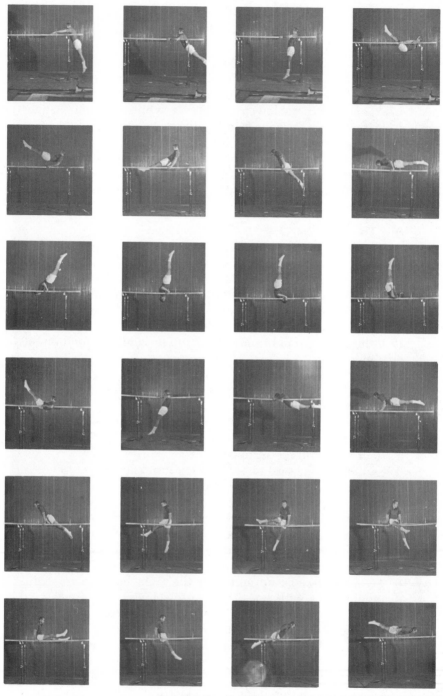

Parallel Bar Routine #3.

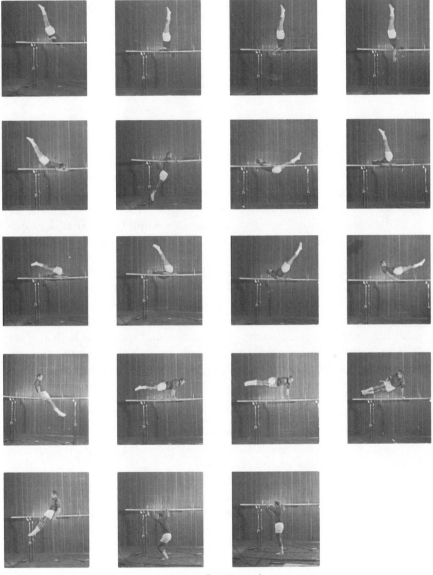

Figure Continued.

CHAPTER 5

THE SIDE HORSE

Maintaining one's body in a support position on the horse requires considerable upper body strength, and most students are relatively weak in this area. Gymnastics in general, and side horse exercises in particular, comprise one of the few physical education activities that emphasize upper body development. For this reason alone, support moves on the side horse are a valuable experience for you.

Instruction on the side horse should begin with the three basic support positions, front (the front of the body against the horse), rear (the rear of the body against the horse), and straddle (the body supported directly over the horse with one leg on either side). In addition to the nomenclature on positions and movements described in Chapter 1, you should understand the terms used to describe movement on the horse. The term "cut," as in "single leg cut," refers to a movement of one or both legs from one side of the horse to the other. This requires lifting one hand and leaning onto the other hand, so that your legs may pass under the lifted hand. The cut may be executed in either a clockwise or counterclockwise direction. Notice that a single leg cut from a front support position results in a straddle, or scissor support position.

The second movement term with which you should be familiar is the word "circle." Circles refer to a movement of one or both legs from one side of the horse to the other and return in one continuous motion. This requires the alternate lifting of one hand and then the other with resultant leaning on the support hand so that your leg or legs may make their circle. Like the cut, this move may be performed either clockwise or counterclockwise.

Finally, you should understand that the horse is divided into three parts: the neck, the saddle, and the croup. Assuming that you always mount from the horse's left side, the neck is always on your left, the croup on your right, and the saddle in the middle. During the performance of a routine, these parts remain in the same position even though you should turn around; however, a second performer may mount from the other side of the horse, and for him the neck is at the other end. In other words, the neck is always designated as being on your left as you mount.

With these terms in mind, you should learn the following skills.

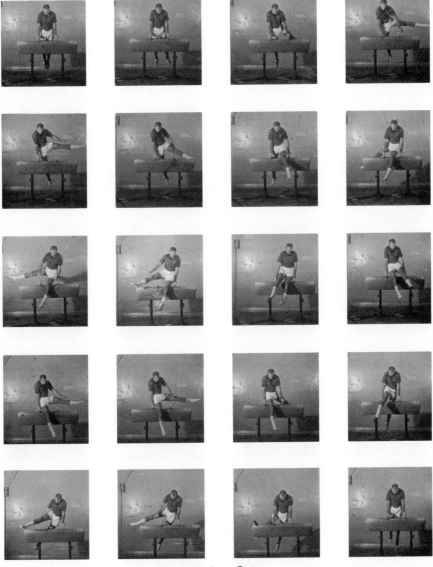

Alternate Leg Cuts.

ALTERNATE LEG CUTS

From a front support in the saddle, cut your left leg CW (clockwise) under your left hand, and then your right leg CCW (counterclockwise) under your right hand. You are now in a rear support position. Next, cut your left leg CCW under your left hand and your right leg CW under your right hand to return to the front support position. Your legs should alternate in their action and the total movement should be continuous and similar to the tick-tock action of a clock pendulum. Remember that, when one hand lifts up to allow a leg cut, your weight must be shifted to the other hand to counterbalance your body. Thus, alternate leg cuts require alternate and opposite weight shifts from arm to arm. These alternate cuts may be performed in the saddle, on the neck, or on the croup.

SINGLE LEG CIRCLE

From a front support position, circle your left leg CW first under your left hand to a scissor position and immediately under your right hand to return to the front support position. Like the alternate leg

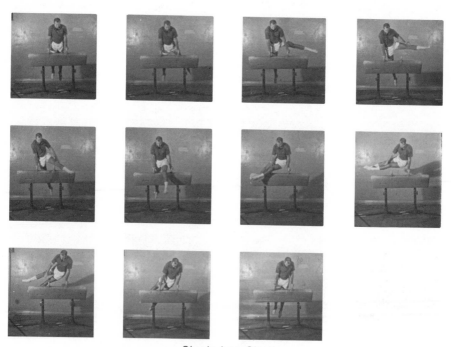

Single Leg Circle.

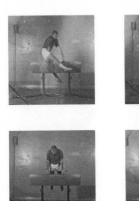
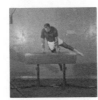

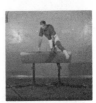
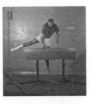
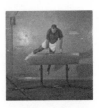
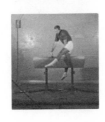
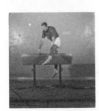

Feint and Swing.

cuts, the movement should be continuous, but there is no tick-tock action because the other leg remains relatively static. This skill may be performed in any one of four ways: the left leg CW or CCW, or the right leg CW or CCW. It may also be performed on the neck, saddle, or croup. Once again, your weight must shift alternately to your supporting hand.

FEINT AND SWING

Feints are actually counter-moves and are not used in routines, but they are helpful in assisting in gaining momentum and learning new moves. From a front support, swing your right leg around the pommel but do not release your grip with either hand.

From this straddle position swing your right leg CW with a vigorous action which lifts your whole body away from the horse. Now use this momentum to lift your left leg around the pommel (again without lifting your hand) to a feint in the other direction. Practice alternating the right and left feints until one follows smoothly after the other.

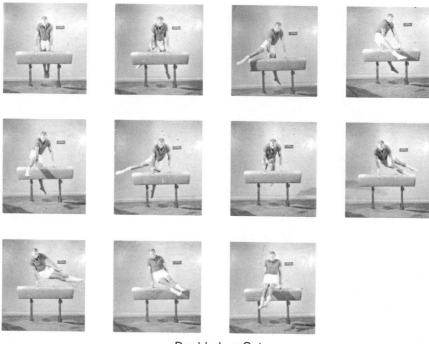

Double Leg Cut.

DOUBLE LEG CUT

This skill is performed like the leg circle, except that both legs are moved simultaneously and only half way around. From a front support position, feint with your right leg and swing it back vigorously; then lean on your right hand and cut both legs under your left hand to a rear support. This is more difficult than the single leg cut because the additional weight of both legs requires that more weight be put on the support hand. Of course, it may be performed in either direction and may also be used as a dismount with the performer landing in a side stand rearways. Note that if your legs are continued around and under the right hand in the same direction, the skill becomes a double leg circle.

ROUTINE #1

Once again continuing with our philosophy that gymnastics should not consist of isolated moves, let us take a look at a simple routine that may be constructed using only the three skills mentioned above.

1. From a side stand frontways at the neck, place your left hand on the neck and your right hand on the left pommel.
2. Jump to front support and cut your left leg under your left hand CW.
3. Swing your right leg over the saddle CCW, but do not release your right hand from the pommel (you are now in a straddle position on the left pommel).
4. Cut your left leg CCW under your left hand and move your left hand from the neck to the left pommel (both hands are now on the left pommel with your right hand in an under grip, your left hand in over grip, and your body in a cross position on horse).
5. Cut your right leg CW over the right pommel and move your right hand to the right pommel (you are now in a front support in the saddle).
6. Cut your left leg CW under your left hand.
7. Swing your right leg CCW over the croup, but do not release your grip on the right pommel (you are now straddling right pommel).
8. Cut your left leg CCW under your left hand and move your left hand to the right pommel (both hands are now on the right pommel with your right hand in an under grip and your left hand in an over grip; your body is in a cross position on the horse).
9. Cut your right leg CW over the croup and move your right hand to the croup (you are now in a front support on the croup).
10. Cut both legs CW under your left hand while leaning hard on your right hand, and push off to a side stand rearways at the croup (you may elect to execute a 1/4 turn CW and push off to a cross stand right at the croup).

This routine sounds most difficult when reading it, but upon consideration of the skills, you will recognize that it is only a combination of the simple moves described earlier in this chapter. Notice that moves 3 through 10 are variations on the alternate leg cuts and result in the performer traveling from the neck to the croup. Such a combination of moves is usually called "alternated leg cut travels."

You can probably complete the routine just described with a couple of hours practice. Notice that as you improve your technique, the movements become easier. This is not the result of an increase in strength, but rather of an improvement in grace and coordination. You are learning to use the momentum developed in one move to assist you in performing another. Keep working toward this goal, for this is the difference between the good and the poor gymnast.

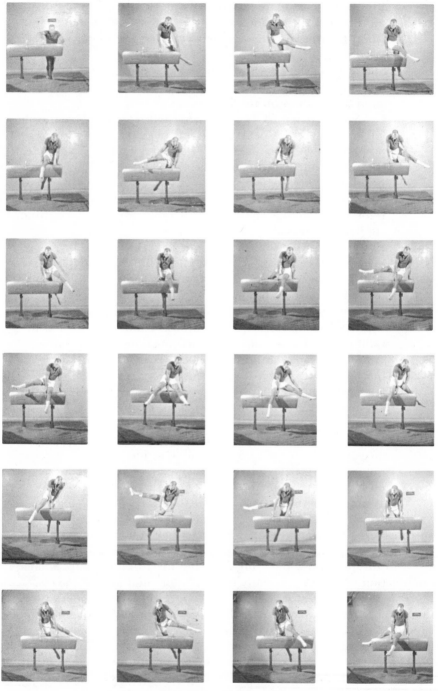

Side Horse Routine #1.

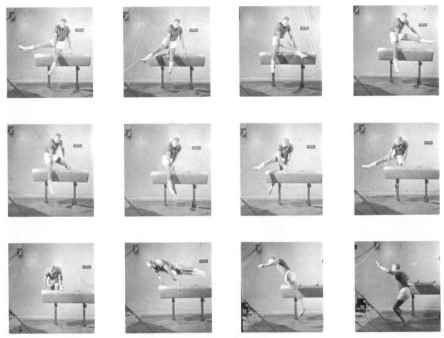

Figure Continued.

SCISSORS

Scissors are the next move you should make. This movement can be described as a cut of both legs at the same time over the same pommel in different directions. Assume you are in a side position straddle in the saddle with your left leg in front and your right leg in the rear. Now swing your legs from side to side without cuts. Let this tick-tock swing continue for several cycles or until you have learned to swing smoothly. Notice that when you swing to the right, the front of your body is leading, and as you swing to the left, the rear of your body is leading. Next swing both legs up to the right again and shift your weight to your left hand. When your legs are at the top of their right swing, release your right hand and switch your left leg to the rear and your right leg to the front, coming back down into a straddle position again.

Notice that you are now in a position to perform another scissor, but this time over the left pommel. If the first one is properly performed, your swing down from the right scissors should assist you in executing the left scissors. Since the front of your body is leading into each of these scissors, the movements are called front scissors right and front scissors left.

If you start in the straddle position with your left leg in front, and

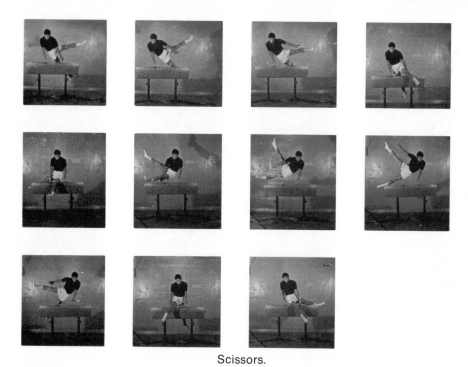

Scissors.

swing your legs up and perform a scissors over the left pommel, then the back of your body would be leading; we call this a reverse scissors. Practice both kinds of scissors until you can repeat at least two fronts in a row and two reverses in a row. You will probably find this a little more difficult than alternate leg cut travels, so don't be discouraged if you do not master it on the first few tries. Keep trying and remember that the single most important factor to remember is to lean on the opposite hand for support while the other hand is raised to allow your legs to pass over the pommel. Additional hints are: keep your knees straight and lift the back leg high.

ROUTINE #2

After you have learned scissors, you should insert them into your basic routine described earlier. Notice that step number 5 brings you to a front support. From here, cut your left leg CW over the left pommel to a straddle position and execute a front scissors right. Cut your left leg CW, then your right leg CW, so that you are now in a straddle position at the saddle with your left leg in front. Now execute a reverse scissors left (over the left pommel). Cut your right leg CW and your left leg CW to return to a straddle with the left leg in front. This

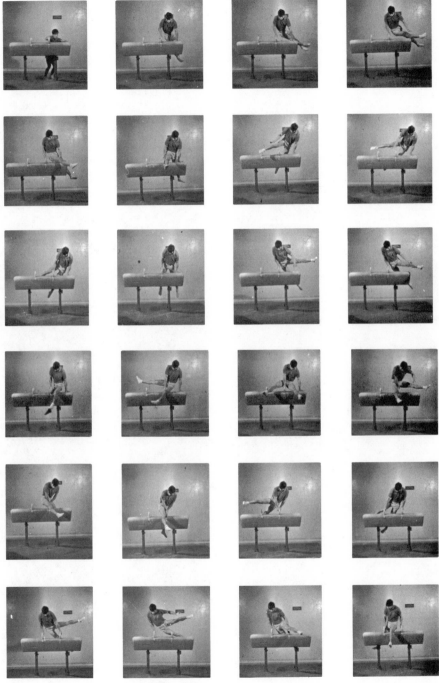

Side Horse Routine #2.

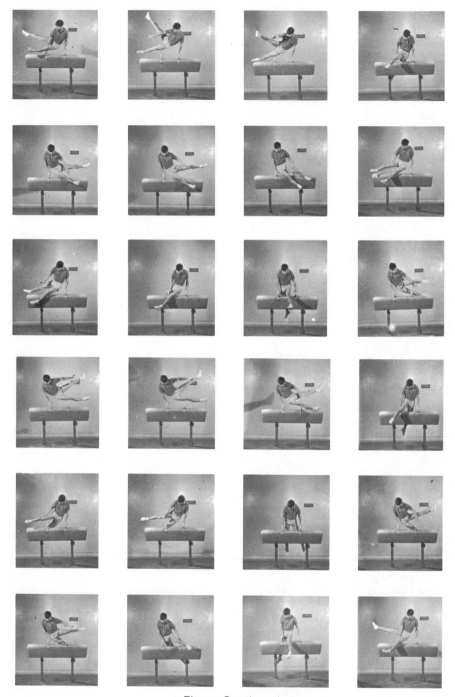

Figure Continued.

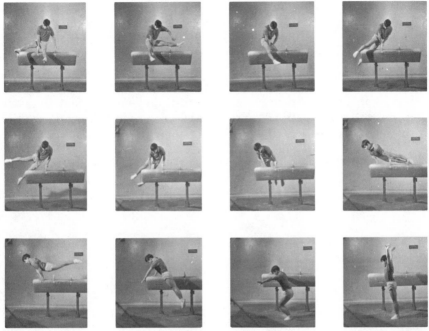

Figure Continued.

is the same position that is described in step number 6. (You may want to review Routine #1 for details of the various moves.) From here, just complete steps number 7 through 10 to finish the routine. In more simple terms, this second routine can be described as follows: From a side stand frontways at the neck,

1. Jump to a front support and cut the left leg clockwise.
2. Alternate leg cut travel to the saddle.
3. Cut your left leg CW over the left pommel and execute a front scissors right.
4. Cut your left leg CW and your right leg CW and execute a rear scissors left.
5. Cut right leg CW and left leg CW.
6. Alternate leg cut travel to the croup.
7. Double leg cut CW over the right pommel to a side stand rearways at the croup. (One quarter turn CW may be added to result in a cross stand right at the croup.)

DOUBLE LEG CIRCLES

The final basic skill you should learn is the double leg circle. This maneuver represents the jumping off point for all intermediate side horse work and is the basis for all advanced skills. To perform a double leg circle, you must swing both legs from one side of the horse, around in a circle under each hand in turn, and back to their original position. Start by performing a feint right and a double leg cut under your left hand. With both legs now in front of the horse, place your left hand back on the left pommel and shift your upper body over the left pommel so that your weight now rests on your left hand. Let your legs continue in their CW circle under your right hand and over the right pommel so that they return to their original position of side support frontways. This double leg circle is most easily performed in the saddle, but may be executed at either the neck or the croup.

This is not an easy maneuver to learn, and it will take much practice to master it. After the feint, you will probably only make it

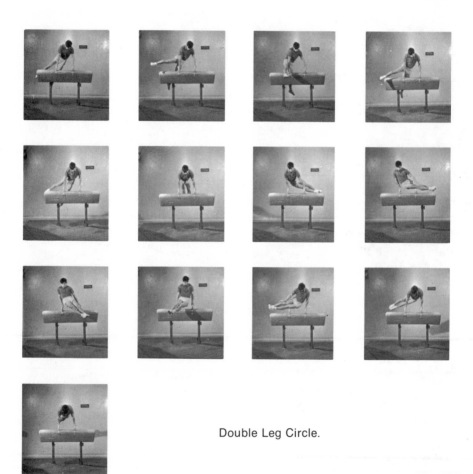

Double Leg Circle.

halfway around on the first few tries. Remember, the weight must be shifted twice in each circle, and the shifts must coincide with the swing of the legs. As you gain skill, try to extend your hips so that your body makes a straight line, and swing from your shoulders. Good side horse performance requires a stretched body and an extended swing.

ROUTINE #3

Like the scissors, double leg circles may be incorporated into the basic routine. After the rear scissors and the CW right and left leg cuts, swing your right leg over the right pommel but do not release your right hand. Then cut your left leg CCW and feint into one or two double leg circles CW. As the legs return to the front support position, cut your left leg CW and complete steps number 7 through 10. The third routine is thus described: From a side stand frontways at the neck,

1. Jump to a front support and cut your left leg clockwise.
2. Alternate leg cut travel to the saddle.
3. Cut your left leg CW over the left pommel and execute a front scissors right.
4. Cut your left leg CW and your right leg CW, and execute a rear scissors left.
5. Cut your right leg CW and your left leg CW.
6. Swing your right leg CCW over the right pommel without release of your right hand, and swing your left leg CCW and feint to one or two double leg circles CW.
7. When you come around to a front support, cut your left leg CW.
8. Alternate leg cut travel to the croup.
9. Double leg cut CW over right pommel to a side stand rearways (or add a one quarter turn CW to a cross stand right at the croup).

This routine contains all of the elements of good side horse work: cuts, circles, front and rear scissors, and travels. It should be performed with continuity and without stops or counter moves. Try to maintain a continual and alternating weight shift from hand to hand and strive to keep your body stretched. With much practice and hard work, this routine can become flowing, smooth, and graceful. Mere completion of the skills is not the ultimate end. They must be performed with elegance and style to accomplish the final objective of "making it look easy."

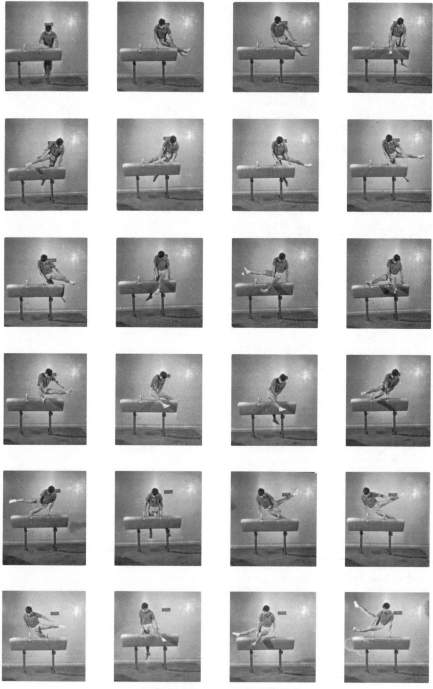

Side Horse Routine #3.

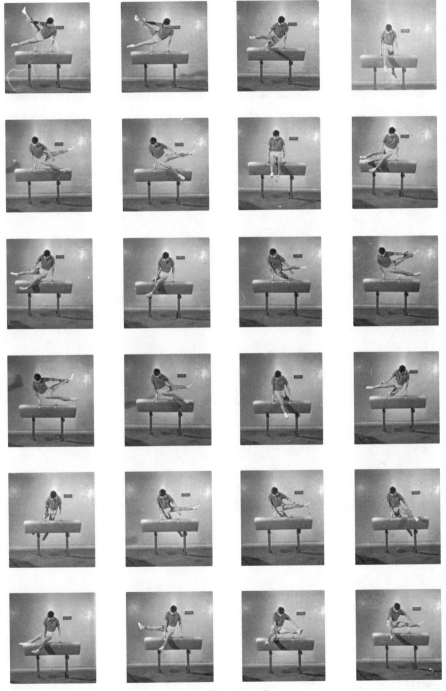

Figure Continued.

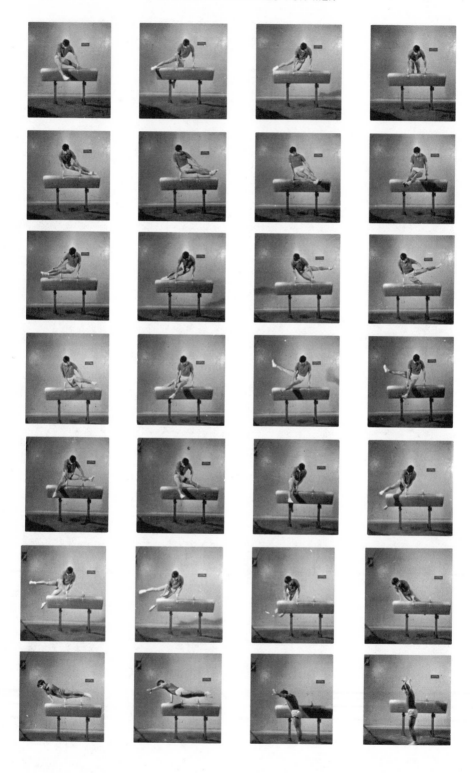

CHAPTER 6

THE HORIZONTAL BAR

Horizontal bars, like parallel bars, are common to most gymnasiums. However, teachers usually neglect them except for testing chinups and teaching a few simple skills such as skin the cat and the bar snap. They are usually very popular out in the sand pit, where interested and talented youngsters learn kips, knee and hock circles, flyaways, uprises, and even giants, without instruction or spotters. Some of these skills are certainly within the range of your ability and can be mastered with the help of your instructor and this book to make performance on the horizontal bar a most enjoyable exercise.

Instruction on horizontal bar should always begin with a few comments on safety. Indeed, this is the proper start for instruction in all events. Safety instruction in all of the hanging and grasping events (parallels, horizontal bars, rings) should include the following three points: grip, chalk, and spotting. They will be discussed here as they pertain to the horizontal bar. The grip should always be of the opposable type; that is, the fingers and thumb should be pointing in opposite directions. Also, with a few exceptions (such as the forward hip circle to cast off), your thumbs should point in the direction of rotation of your body around the bar. This prevents your hands from peeling off the bar as your body swings.

Chalk is a must on the horizontal bar, as it assists in maintaining a good grip on the apparatus. Contrary to some opinion, chalk does not reduce the possibility of blisters; rather, it increases the coefficient of friction between the hands and the bar, thereby reducing the possibility of slipping.

Both instructor and pupils should practice spotting. (Review Chapter 2 for detailed information on safety.) Once you are aware of the basic safety aspects, you may begin practice on the following elementary skills. (The bar is usually placed about eye level at first and may be moved up for some skills as indicated later in this chapter.)

BAR SNAP

From a side stand frontways with your hands in an over grip, jump upward to about a half straight arm support. During the jump, bend your hips and place your shins or ankles under and near the opposite side of the bar. As your body swings forward and under the bar, vigorously extend your hips and push away from the bar with your arms, shooting your legs and body into an arch, resulting in a side stand rearways.

Upon mastery of the snap from a stand, the action may be initiated from a front leaning support above the bar. From this position push the bar down toward your thighs and then rotate backward while sliding the bar down your legs from thighs to shins or ankles. The skill is then completed as a normal bar snap. It can be used as a dismount at the conclusion of a routine, or it can be used as a testing device by measuring the distance between the bar and your heels on landing.

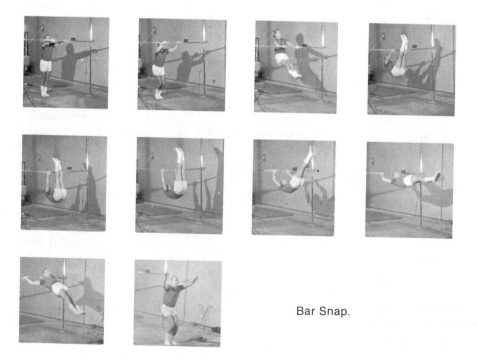

Bar Snap.

PULL OVER

This common skill is excellent for developing strength in your arms, shoulders, and abdominal area. It is a convenient beginning move because it can be learned with the bar at eye level first and then with the bar at hanging height. At eye level, with an over grip, begin by swinging one leg under and over the other side of the bar. At the same time, execute a chinup and hold yourself in this position until your hips contact the top of the bar. As you bring your legs together, you should attempt to contact the bar as far up on the pelvis as possible so that you may continue your rotation around to a front leaning support. Shifting your hands to a position above the bar during this final step will assist in attaining the full support. Spotters may assist by standing on the sides and placing one hand on your lower back, the other on the back of your thigh at the start. They should then shift both hands to the shoulder and forearm after the hips are on the bar to help in the final rise to support.

On a tall bar, the student must first chin himself, then hold the chin position while he pulls his legs up and over the bar. As a practice routine, this skill may be combined with the bar snap in one continuous action.

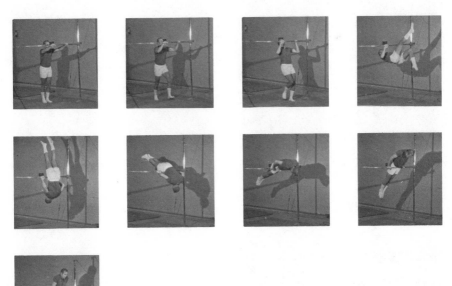

Pull Over.

BACKWARD HIP CIRCLE

The hip circle is similar to the pullover in its final stage, but starts from a front leaning support on the bar. You should first learn this skill by swinging your legs under the bar and then casting slightly backward so that your hips disengage the bar by about four to six inches. This feinting action sets your body for proper execution. As your hips again engage the bar after the feint, your knees and hips are both flexed so that your body folds up around the bar. Now shift your hands under and around the bar so that you can push down to help yourself return to the support position. Contact between your hips and the bar must be maintained or your body will fall under the bar and you will be unable to make a complete circle. Spotters can prevent this and assist in the rotation by using their hands in a manner similar to that used in the pull over. As your legs swing under the bar, one hand is placed on the back of your thigh to assist rotation and the other is placed behind your lower back to prevent your hips from falling away. As the movement is completed, the hands can shift to your shoulder and forearm to help maintain the support position.

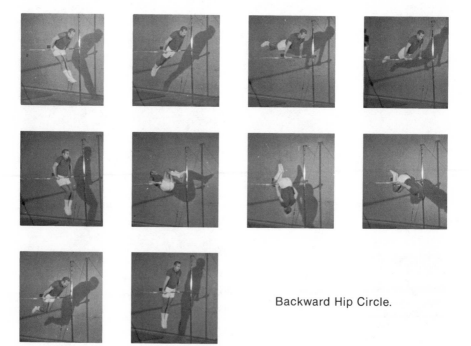

Backward Hip Circle.

ROUTINE #1

With these three skills mastered, you are ready for Routine #1. It is quite short and simple but it prepares you for later skills. With the bar at eye level, combine your skills in the order listed:
1. From a side stand frontways with over grip, pull over to front leaning support.
2. Feint and execute a backward hip circle, returning to front leaning support, and . . .
3. Swing back and under the bar to a bar snap dismount to a side stand rearways.

After a couple of tries, eliminate the feint and make all three moves continuous, without counterswings.

CAST WITH HALF TURN TO MIXED GRIP

This is a transition maneuver that contains a 180 degree turn and is executed in a manner similar to the bar snap from above the bar. Begin by casting your legs under the bar from a front support position just like the beginning of a bar snap, except that your legs cast slightly to the left instead of straight ahead. As they cast diagonally left, your right hand is released and your body executes a one-half turn counterclockwise around your left hand, which is still in contact with the bar. Your right hand regrasps on the other side of your left hand and your body swings forward in mixed grip with your left hand under and your right hand over. You should be careful to keep your hips close to the bar during preliminary rotation so that the turn and the extension of the hips can coincide in a smooth movement allowing your right hand to regrasp before your body reaches the midpoint on the forward swing. The entire maneuver can be executed in reverse direction.

Spotters use hand positions similar to those used for the back hip circle, but must be ready to move their hands as your body turns and still maintain control. To properly execute the cast with one half turn, the bar must be high enough to allow the performer to swing under it with a relatively straight body. Eight or ten inches above the head should be sufficient.

SINGLE KNEE RISE

With an over grip and one knee hooked on the bar between the hands, swing back and forth under the bar. On one of the backward swings, kick your free leg down and backward and at the same time lean over the bar with your head and shoulders. After a quick shift of

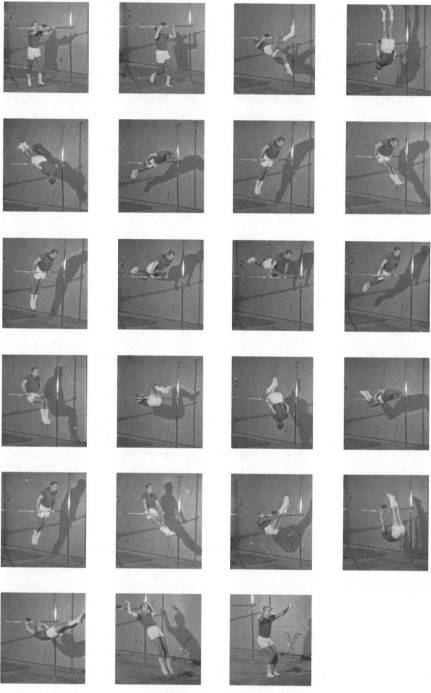

Horizontal Bar Routine #1.

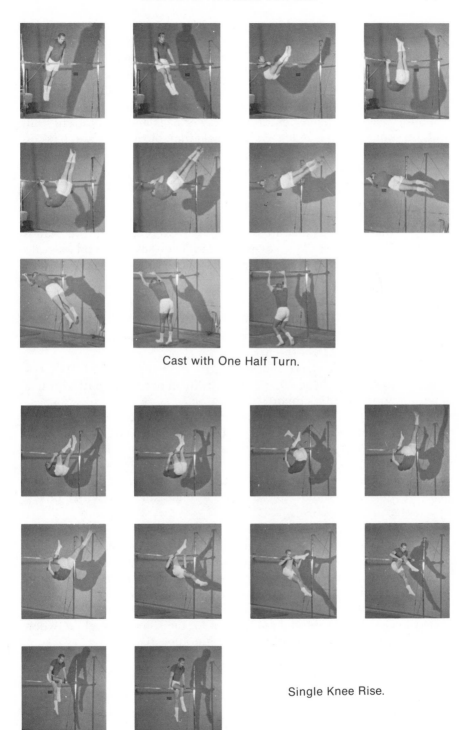

Cast with One Half Turn.

Single Knee Rise.

your hands to a position above the bar, balance in a support position with one leg in front and one leg behind the bar. The kick of your free leg is the action that results in correct performance of this skill, and care should be taken to keep this leg straight and make the kick correspond to the backward swing of your body. Without a strong coordinated kick, the skill cannot be performed properly. Spotters should place one hand behind your lower back and the other in front of the knee of your free leg. As you kick, they push down and back on your knee and lift your lower back. The spotter's knee hand should then shift to the other side of the bar and hold your upper arm as you complete the movement to prevent you from falling forward over the top of the bar.

After you learn this basic knee mount, try it from an underswing. As your body swings forward, one foot is passed between your hands so that the knee can hook over the bar. Then, as your body swings back, your free leg kicks and you ride up and over the bar.

ROUTINE #2

Now you are ready for a second routine which is longer and more complicated than the first one.
1. From a side stand frontways, with the bar about 6 to 10 inches above your head and your hands in an over grip, pull over to a front leaning support.
2. Continue backwards to a backward hip circle.
3. Cast under and forward with one half turn counterclockwise around your left hand, regrasping with your right hand in a mixed grip.
4. Swing forward and pass your right leg between your hands and under the bar and execute a single knee rise with a mixed grip.
5. Without releasing your left hand, turn your body 180 degrees counterclockwise, releasing and regrasping your right hand in an over grip on the other side of your body.
6. Swing your left leg over the bar to a front leaning support and bar snap dismount to a side stand rearways.

This routine should be performed without stops. Try to keep your knees straight throughout, except for the stoop through between your hands in preparation for the single knee rise.

KIP

The kip on the horizontal bar is one of the most popular skills in gymnastics. It is similar to the kips learned in the other events, but on the horizontal bar it is combined with an underswing, so that the timing is very important. Because of the underswing, the bar must be high enough to prevent your feet from dragging on the mat. From an underswing with an over grip, swing as smoothly as possible so that your body does not bounce or jerk on the bar. As you pass the center on one of the forward swings, begin bending your hips so that on the end of the forward swing, your ankles are almost in contact with the bar. Now let your backswing begin slightly and then pull the bar along your legs past your shin, knees and thighs until it reaches your hips. This sliding of the bar along your legs coincides with your backward swing so that the two actions conclude simultaneously. This combined action should raise you above the bar to a front leaning support. When you approach this position, lean your head over the bar to complete the action.

Contrary to some belief, the action on the kip is not a kick away from the bar, but rather an extension of the hip joint so that you pull the bar along your legs. Think of the action as being upside down while you pull your pants on with your knees straight. As mentioned before, the hard part is not the pull, but the timing of the pull and the backswing. Study the pictures and then have the spotters assist you by pushing on your lower back to help you attain the full support position.

FORWARD CAST

This is not a part of the routine, except that it allows you to acquire the swing needed to perform other skills. It is especially helpful in attaining the necessary swing for the rear uprise. It may be performed with either an over or under grip, or even a mixed grip, depending upon which skill is to follow.

From a hang under the bar with a very small swing, chin yourself at the conclusion of one of the back swings and raise your feet under and on the other side of the bar as in a bar snap. Now extend your feet and legs upward on the other side of the bar at about 30 degrees or higher. At the same time, push away from the bar with your hands but continue to maintain your grip. This places your body in an extended position above the bar and allows for a large backswing. (See page 79.)

REAR SWING RISE

The rear swing rise or uprise is another method of mounting or getting up on the bar. This skill requires a larger underswing and

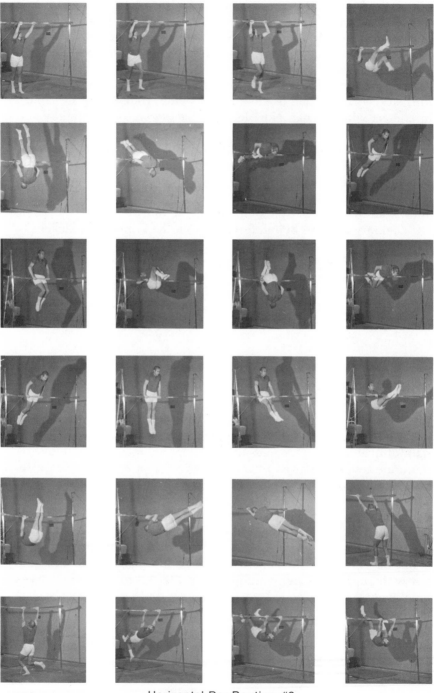

Horizontal Bar Routine #2.

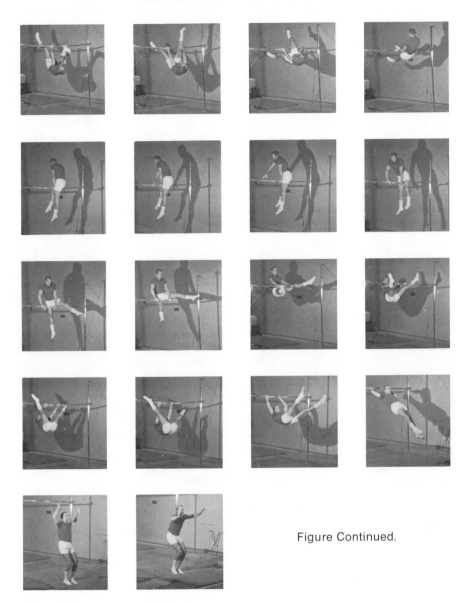

Figure Continued.

should be performed after a forward cast. With an over hand grip, as your body swings backward, wait until you pass the midpoint; then push down hard on the bar with your elbows straight. As your body rises on the back swing, the bar should be drawn toward your hips so that you attain the full support position with straight elbows. This push and swing must be coordinated as in the kip so that they complement each other in raising your body above the bar. As your

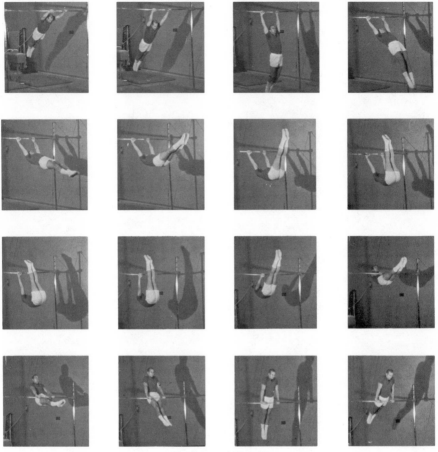

Horizontal Bar Kip.

hips come in contact with the bar, immediately execute a backward hip circle to absorb the shock of contact with the bar.

ROUTINE #3

This routine will be the same as Routine #2 except for the mount. You may substitute either the kip or the rear uprise for the pull over as described in Routine #2. If the kip is used, a feint will be necessary between the kip and the back hip circle. If you use the uprise, the back hip circle will follow smoothly. For this reason the routine will be described with the rear uprise as the mount. Raise the bar high enough so that your feet will not drag on the mat.

 1. From a side stand frontways, jump to a hang with an over grip.

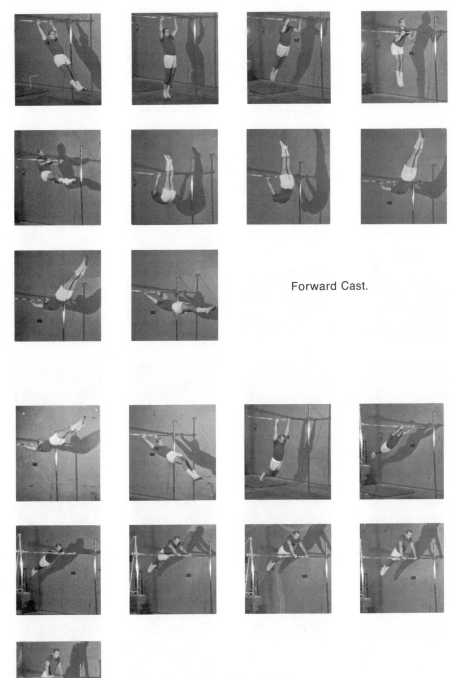

Forward Cast.

Rear Swing Rise.

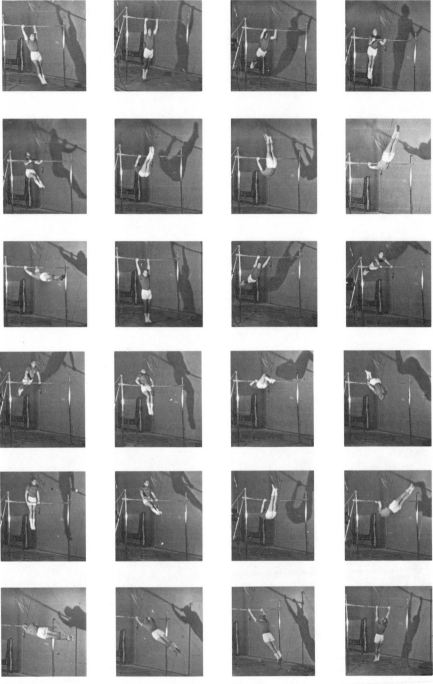

Horizontal Bar Routine #3.

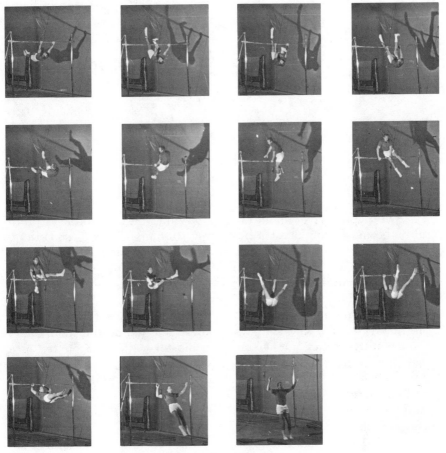

Figure Continued.

2. Cast forward and swing backward to a rear uprise. Continue around the bar to a. . .
3. Reverse hip circle, and further continue around and under the bar to a. . .
4. Cast with one half turn, to a forward swing with mixed grip.
5. Stoop your right leg under the bar and between your hands to a single knee rise.
6. Rotate 180 degrees around your left hand, disengage your left leg, and. . .
7. Bar snap forward to a side stand rearways.

This routine represents a combination of beginning and intermediate skills on the horizontal bar. Strive for perfection of these before you advance to more difficult moves. Remember, the goal of gymnastics is not to perform skills in isolation, but to combine them into a well coordinated routine that "makes it look easy."

CHAPTER 7

THE TRAMPOLINE

Of all the apparatus in the gymnasium, the trampoline is probably the most popular with beginning students. There is something exhilarating about flying through the air, free for a few moments from the otherwise ever-present pull of gravity. In addition, the unique concept of landing on seats, backs, and stomachs rather than feet offers a feeling not attainable elsewhere.

Beginning trampoline is probably one of the safest events. There are many simple, safe skills that can be learned on the trampoline. You could practice for an entire semester without even trying a complete somersault. This may not be desirable, since somersaults themselves are not particularly dangerous, but the point being made is that there are many basic skills, and particularly combinations of skills or routines, that can challenge you without offering the element of danger.

Frequently, instructors and students feel that to perform properly on trampoline, great height must be attained. This is not so. All of the skills described in this chapter and many more can be successfully performed with only one or two feet of bounce.

The trampoline is popular with many students because they can achieve success without possessing the upper body strength required in other events. Students who are relatively unsuccessful on parallel bars, horizontal bar, and rings may make considerable progress on the trampoline. Rebound tumbling, as it is sometimes called, also offers a unique opportunity to combine skills into simple routines, since the strength factor is reduced and the skills lend themselves naturally to continuation of movement.

Before learning to bounce on the trampoline, you should be made aware of some special spotting techniques. You should never bounce without spotters, and spotters must pay strict attention to their performer. If the performer comes close to the edge, spotters should hold up their hands and attempt to push the performer back onto the bed. Attempts to catch the student as he falls usually result in both the performer and the spotter collapsing to the ground. Consequently, pushing him back on the bed is the more accepted technique.

Initial instruction should also include a comment about getting on and off the trampoline and simple bouncing. Sitting on the frame and then rolling onto the bed for mounting, and the opposite for dismounting, is the safest method. When you begin to bounce, stay in the middle and land with your feet shoulder width apart. Circle your arms so they come up in front on the up bounce and down at your sides on the down bounce. Focus your eyes on the springs or frame at the end of the bed. This will give you the proper head position, as well as something to spot so that your orientation in the air may be maintained.

In this chapter, only a few of the basic skills will be discussed, but it is felt that they will be most beneficial to you and would fit together best for simple routines. The first four skills are called the "basic four," since they train you to land on all parts of your body. This ability will be most beneficial in later learning, as it will help you land safely when you fail to complete a more difficult move.

HANDS AND KNEES DROP

This skill is performed just as the name implies. In the landing position your back is parallel to the bed. Your weight should be

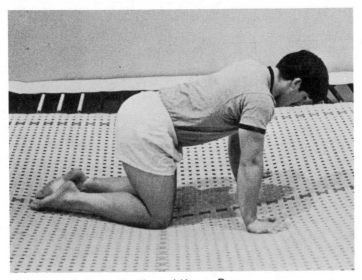

Hands and Knees Drop.

equally placed on all four limbs. This avoids the "rocking horse" effect and provides for a straight rebound to return to your feet. Begin by bouncing in the landing position until some control is obtained; then start from your feet and rebound back to your feet after landing. Later you may eliminate your hands and land on your knees only. When doing this, keep your back vertical, with your knees, hips, and shoulders in line.

SEAT DROP

Begin this move by sitting on the bed with your hips on the cross in the webbing. Your knees should be straight and the back of your legs from your heels to your hips should be in contact with the bed. Place your palms down on the bed beside your hips for balance. The ease of this skill surprises some beginners, since, when performed correctly, you will bounce back to your feet with little or no effort.

FRONT DROP

The front drop also begins with the assumption of the landing position before attempting the entire move. Your hips should be directly over the cross on the bed, your knees held slightly bent, and your elbows bent at 90 degrees with your forearms flat on the bed so that the backs of your hands are directly in front of your face. This is

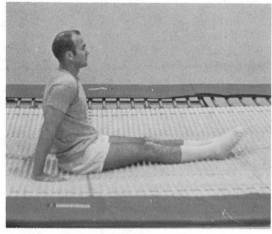

Seat Drop.

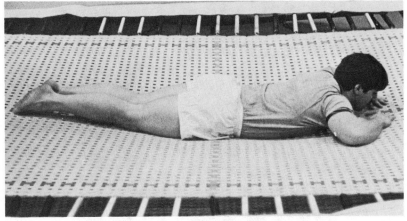

Front Drop.

the landing position, and all parts of the anterior surface of your body, except your face, should contact the bed simultaneously. After assuming the landing position, your first attempt should be from a hands and knees position. With a small bounce, extend your legs backward, your arms forward and contact the bed on your front; then return on the *first* rebound to your hands and knees.

Later, a larger bounce on your hands and knees can precede the landing. You may then progress from feet to hands and knees, to front, to feet; and and finally, from feet to front, to feet. This progression should be flexible so that your progress may be at a rate at which you feel competent.

BACK DROP

Again, to build confidence, you should assume the landing position first so that proper contact with the bed is assumed. Your hips should be over the cross with your legs raised to the vertical position. Your entire back from your shoulders to your hips should be flat on the mat with the weight distributed equally, but the back of your head should not touch the mat. Your arms should be extended in front of your chest for balance. Two methods are suggested for learning this skill. The first requires that you bounce to your back after performing a bent knee seat drop. This allows you to land on your back from a lower bounce and may also assist you in attaining the proper landing position. Upon landing, extend your hips vigorously in coordination with the spring of the bed and rebound back to your feet.

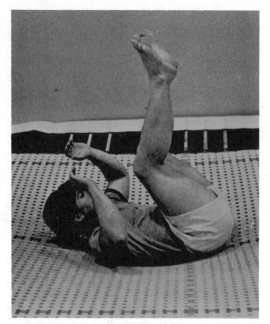

Back Drop.

An alternate method begins by standing on the bed while holding an imaginary beachball in your hands with your arms extended forward about chest high. Then raise one leg and attempt to kick the imaginary ball up to the ceiling. The vigorous kick will force you off balance so that you fall to the bed in the back drop position. The leg upon which you are standing should be kept straight to ensure proper landing and should join the kicking leg in the air so that they are together when your back contacts the bed. Later you may kick with both legs to complete the skill. The rebound to a stand is the same as with the first method. Sometimes you may feel a snap in your neck as you land. This is due to landing with most of the weight on your hips while your shoulders are suspended off the mat. Laying your head back a little farther or raising your legs harder usually corrects this common error.

ROUTINE #1

Now that you have mastered the basic form, you are ready for your first routine. This simple routine consists of a combination of these skills in the following order:

1. From a small bounce in the middle of the bed, drop to your hands and knees.

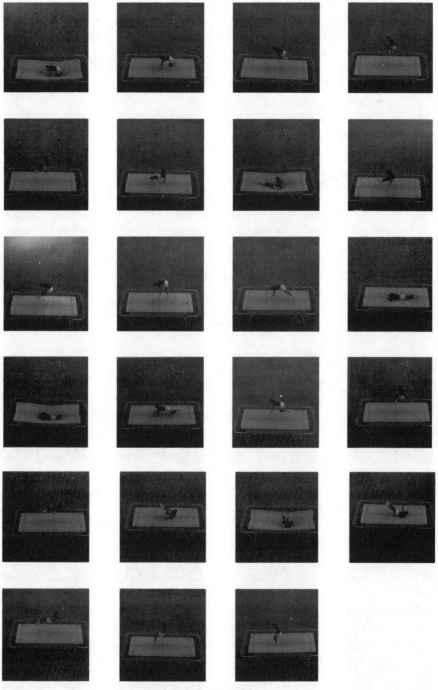

Trampoline Routine #1.

2. Raise your head and straighten your legs to a seat drop.
3. Push with your hands and rotate forward to a front drop.
4. Push with your hands and rotate backward to a back drop.
5. Bounce to your feet.

When you first attempt this routine, bounce on your feet between each skill, but later eliminate these intermediate bounces. To go from your front to your back, push with your hands, look up at the ceiling and snap your knees straight just as you leave the bed after the front drop.

SWIVEL HIPS

This skill consists of a seat drop, a 180 degree turn, and another seat drop without intermediate touching of the mat. Throughout the move, your legs should be kept straight and your feet should follow the line that runs down the long axis of the bed. Bringing your feet around the side in a semi-tuck position is a common error and should be eliminated. The first step in learning consists of a seat drop properly executed and a stand with 90 degree turn. Upon rebounding from the seat drop, push off the mat with your hands, then

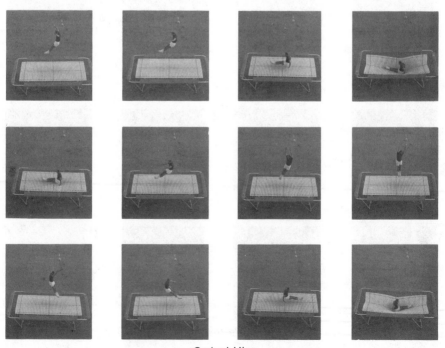

Swivel Hips.

extend them over your head and look in the direction of the turn. Your hips should be extended from the sitting to the standing position, and your body should execute a one quarter turn so that you are standing sideways on the bed with your hands over your head. This same movement should be then repeated with a 180 degree turn so that your body is facing the opposite direction from that in which it started.

Throughout this move you should keep your legs straight and directly under your body. Finally, after completion of the one half turn, you execute another seat drop and sit facing the other way without touching the mat. A slight forward lean on the initial landing position may assist you in making the final seat drop.

HALF TWIST TO FRONT DROP, OR ONE HALF AIRPLANE

Sometimes this maneuver is called an airplane, but it is preferable to include the prefix "one half," since it contains only a one half twist. This helps differentiate it from the full airplane, which contains a full twist. The move actually consists of a back drop with one half twist, landing on the front, and should be performed without

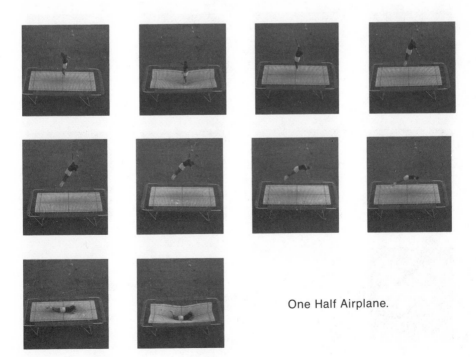

One Half Airplane.

a bounce when it is first attempted. Begin by falling back with a relatively straight body (not with a kick as described in the back drop) and, as you fall, turning 180 degrees and landing in a front drop. After a few practices without bounce, you may gradually build up height. When confidence is obtained, your arms may be extended to the sides during the turn and you can "fly" around, giving the airplane effect. Control can be improved by looking and pointing the lead arm directly at the intended landing spot.

ONE HALF TURNTABLE

This movement is essentially a front drop, a 180 degree turn around the depth axis, and another front drop. The front of your body faces the mat throughout the movement. As you rebound from your first front drop, push to the side with your arms and look sideways around your shoulder. Pulling your knees into a tuck position accelerates the turn, which culminates in another front drop with your body facing in the other direction. Learning may be facilitated by practicing the one quarter turntable first to master the fundamentals. A full turntable would consist of a 360 degree turn from front drop to front drop.

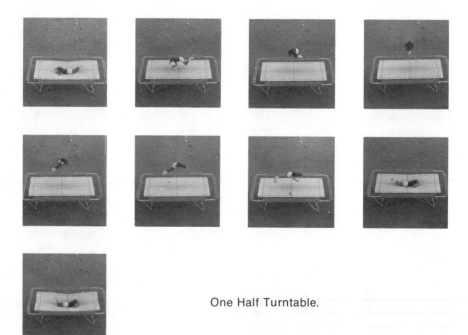

One Half Turntable.

ROUTINE #2

These new skills may now be combined into many different patterns. You may want to experiment with different combinations; however, the following order is suggested for your first try.

1. One half airplane.
2. Turntable.
3. Bounce to feet.
4. Seat to swivel hips.
5. Bounce to feet.

Remember that the most important factor in performing this or any other routine is the smoothness with which the skills flow together. The trampoline offers a unique opportunity to accentuate this flow. Merely performing the skills one at a time does not satisfy the objective of performing smoothly and in a well coordinated action.

FULL AIRPLANE

The full airplane begins in the same manner as the one half airplane, and you are advised not to attempt this new skill until you have completely mastered the more elementary one. The full airplane ends in a back drop, and should be performed so that the landing position is the same as a properly executed back drop.

After your take off into the air as in a one half airplane, look at the mat and begin descending as if you were going to land on your front. Then take your trailing arm (right arm if you are turning clockwise) and pull it across your chest while turning your head in the direction of the turn to look at the ceiling. This will spin your body around the length axis so that you will have completed a full turn. (See page 93).

CRADLE

Before you can learn to cradle, you must learn to perform a back drop to a front drop. Neither of these skills is new to you, but the combination may prove to be a little difficult. Practice it until you can do it with ease and agility. Then, as you are coming off your back and have passed the midpoint (extended vertically in the air) and are beginning the front drop, pull one of your arms (preferably the same one you used in the full airplane) across your chest and look in the same direction toward the ceiling. This action of pulling the arm and looking with your head will turn you around, so that you land on your back instead of your front. You can see that a cradle is just a

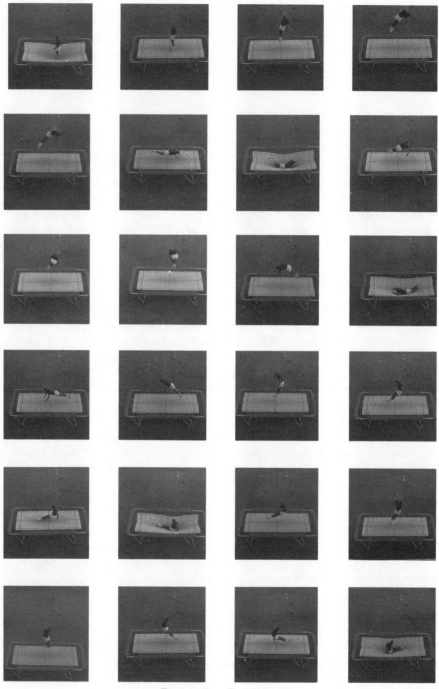

Trampoline Routine #2.

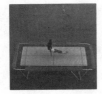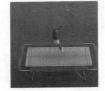

Figure Continued.

back drop to another back drop with a one half turn in between. Remember this method of turning, because it is used in many different gymnastics skills. (See page 94.)

FRONT SOMERSAULT

The front somersault on the trampoline is relatively easy to learn because it can be broken down into many component skills. You have already learned the hands and knees drop, the back drop, and the seat drop. Now you can use these skills to help you master the front somersault. First do a hands and knees drop and bounce over to a back drop. As you rebound from the hands and knees drop, tuck your head under your body so that your chin is on your chest and

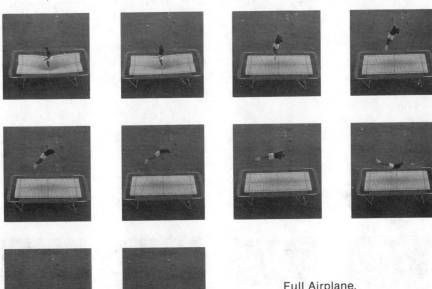

Full Airplane.

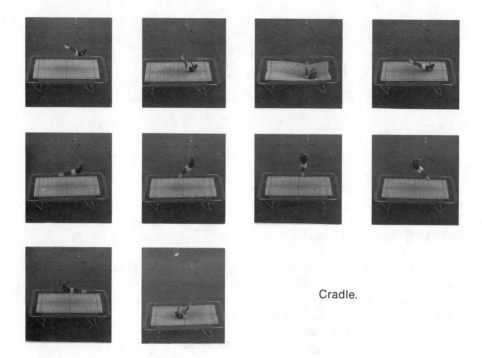

Cradle.

bring your knees up tight to your chest. Then land on your back and rebound to your feet. Practice this until you can do it with complete control.

After you have mastered the hands and knees to back drop, try turning over a little farther and doing a hands and knees to seat drop. This requires a tighter tuck, faster spin, and more control, as you

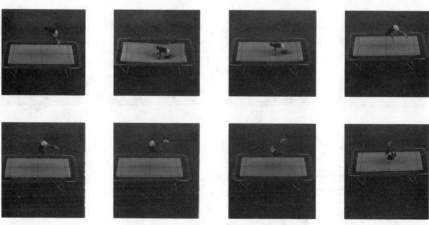

Hands and Knees to Back Drop.

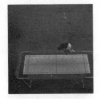
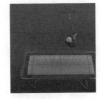
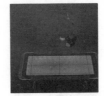

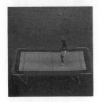

Knees to Feet Front Somersault.

must come out of the tuck and open up to a seat drop and then rebound to your feet.

The third step in the progression involves the same start, but this time you turn all the way over and land on your feet. A slightly higher bounce may be needed to make it all the way around and you may want to take off from your knees only. Land with your feet about shoulder width apart, and be prepared to catch your entire body

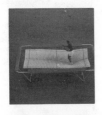
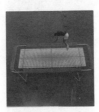
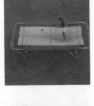
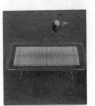

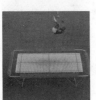

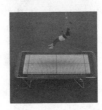
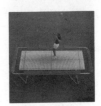

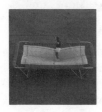

Front Somersault.

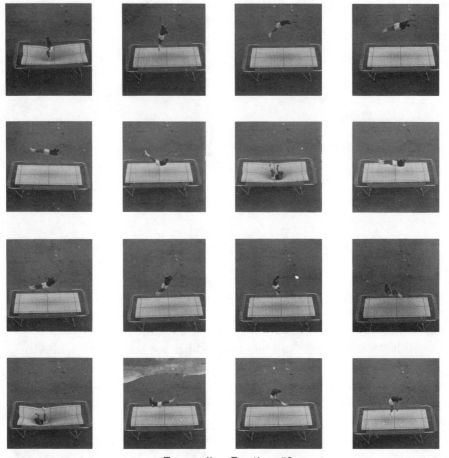

Trampoline Routine #3.

weight when you land. If you do not make it all the way around, just land on your back or seat as previously practiced.

Finally you may eliminate the hands and knees take-off and bounce directly from your feet. When you start from your feet, first practice landing on your back, then on your seat, and finally on your feet. This final step, the feet to feet front somersault, represents the culmination of the progression you have been following. If you find yourself developing some bad habits during the progression, such as traveling too much or turning to the side as you somersault, go back to the beginning and work on a more simple part until you solve your problem. Then progress further until you have completed all of the steps.

There are many other skills on the trampoline which are of the same relative difficulty as the ones you have learned. However,

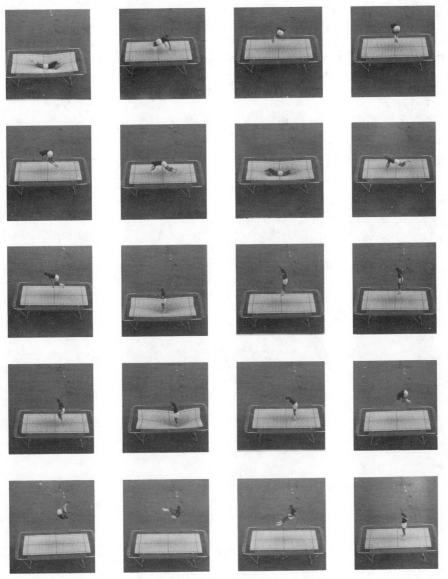

Figure Continued.

remember that the mastery of single skills is not our objective. Rather, we are trying to combine our skills into routines. The skills you have learned represent enough of a repertoire to make up many routines, and you are encouraged to combine them into many different patterns. Try this third one as a starter and then branch out on your own.

ROUTINE #3

This routine combines the final three skills you have learned with some of the earlier ones. Try it in parts first, or add a foot bounce between the difficult combinations as you learn, but strive to perform it eventually without intermediate bounces in a smooth manner.

1. Full airplane, to land on your back.
2. Cradle.
3. Bounce to front drop.
4. Turntable; bounce to feet.
5. One additional foot bounce (optional).
6. Front somersault to feet landing.

By placing the above skills in different order, or by adding additional moves, the difficulty of the routine can be varied.

Practice on your own routines, but remember that difficulty should never be increased at the expense of proper execution.

You should always try to "make it look easy."

CHAPTER 8

THE RINGS

The rings are probably the most difficult event you will encounter, because a great deal of upper body strength is required. Being unstable and free moving, they require that you not only support your own body weight, but also control movement of the apparatus and hold it in position while you perform. At the beginning of your gymnastics experience, you may not have the strength to accomplish this task, so it is advised that the other events be learned first in order to develop your strength.

Like the horizontal bar, the rings are a hanging and swinging apparatus; therefore, all of the safety precautions, such as chalking of the hands, proper grip, and spotting, mentioned in previous chapters are appropriate here (review Chapter 2 for details of these precautions).

The rings should be placed at about eye level at the beginning. This will assist you in mounting, since the apparatus is low enough to enable you to jump to a support position. Later, as your strength improves, the rings may be raised so that the support position must be attained by the use of some skill other than jumping, such as a kip, pull to support (muscle up), or rear swing rise (snap rise or uprise).

BASIC STRENGTH SKILLS

Begin your workouts on rings by practicing some of the more simple strength skills such as chinups with knees bent, straight arm supports, hanging L's and support L's, and the tuck inverted hang. The last skill is performed by raising your legs above your head and between your arms so that your body is supported in an upside down tuck position. Spotters should stand almost underneath to support your upper and lower back. Begin by descending the same way you ascended, but later try going down the opposite way (counterclockwise) until your feet touch the mats. After touching, release the rings and stand up. This completes what is commonly referred to as a simple "skin the cat."

SKIN THE CAT

Upon mastery of the tuck inverted hang and the simple "skin the cat," try the pike and straight body inverted hang. The pike inverted hang is similar to a tuck inverted hang except that, after your body is upside down, the knee joint is extended placing your body in a pike position. From this position, if you were to straighten your hips, you would be in a straight body inverted hang. When you are first attempting to perform these maneuvers, the rings may have a tendency to wobble, but this can be corrected by pressing the rings against the sides of your body to give them more stability.

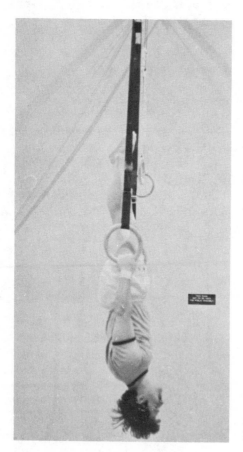

Straight Body Inverted Hang.

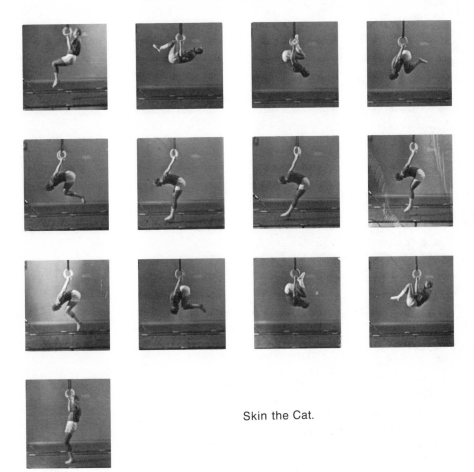

Skin the Cat.

Now try to complete the "skin the cat" by pulling to a tuck inverted hang and continuing on until your feet touch the mat; then, without releasing your grip, pull your feet and legs back over your head in the opposite direction until you return to a tuck inverted hang. You may need help from spotters to get back, or you may have to jump off the mat to get started, but a correct "skin the cat" requires that you bring your toes one inch from the mat and then pull them back up and over without assistance or a jump.

STANDING INLOCATE

The standing inlocate is accomplished by taking a grip on the rings and then moving them with straight arms to the sides of the body. With the rings out to the sides, rotate your arms forward with

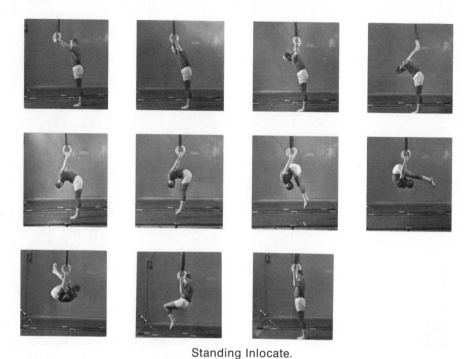

Standing Inlocate.

thumbs down and bring them together again behind your back. During this rotation your head is tucked forward so that your chin contacts your chest. You will now find yourself in the "standing inlocate" position, ready to pull your legs back over your head.

STANDING DISLOCATE

The opposite of the standing inlocate, and another very useful skill when performing routines, is the standing dislocate. The term "dislocate" may cause you some apprehension. When properly performed, this maneuver gives the appearance of dislocating the shoulder, but in reality the arms are simply rotating around. Begin by performing the first half of "skin the cat" until your feet touch the mat. At this point stand up by raising your head and moving the rings from behind your back, out to the side and around to the front. The rings will turn in a direction opposite to that of the inlocate (backwards, or thumbs up), but in the dislocate this occurs naturally and you will automatically turn them in the right direction. As you master the standing dislocate, increase the tempo of the maneuver so that it is performed in one continuous action without a stop as your feet

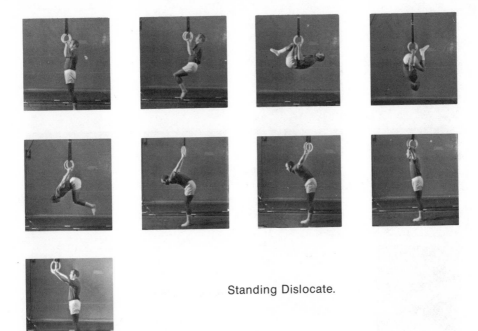

Standing Dislocate.

touch the mat. To accomplish this, begin by lifting your head and moving the rings to the side before your feet touch; then as they touch, complete the action smoothly without a stop.

DISLOCATE TO STAND

This is the next step in learning a true dislocate. Begin from a pike inverted hang and extend your hips vigorously, shooting your feet backward at about a 45 degree angle from the horizontal. At the same time, raise your head rapidly and move your arms out to the side with your elbows straight. As your feet come down and contact the mat, the skill is completed by bringing your hands around to the front and raising your head to a complete standing position. This action is the beginning of the actual dislocate skill. Timing is important here, and much practice will be required before mastery; however, this is an essential skill for later performance on high rings.

ROLL TO INVERTED HANG

The inverted hang position may be attained from above the rings as well as from below, as you have already learned. Once you can

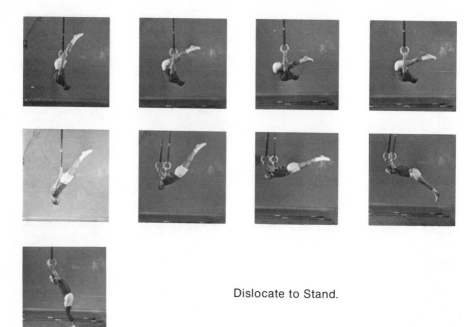

Dislocate to Stand.

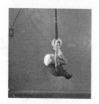

support yourself above the rings, it is a relatively easy maneuver to lower yourself backward or forward to an inverted hang. Rolling backward or counterclockwise is easiest, so begin from the support position by bringing your knees up to your chest and bending your elbows. Now tilt your head back and pull your knees up and over your body until you come to rest in a tuck inverted hang.

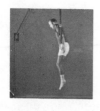
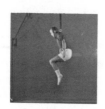
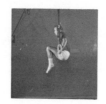
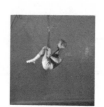

Roll Backward to Inverted Hang.

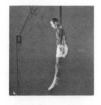 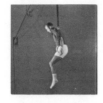 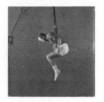 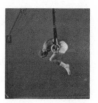

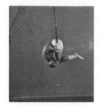 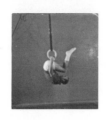

Roll Forward to Inverted Hang.

Spotters may assist you by placing their hands on your upper and lower back to help you rotate, as well as to slow down the roll.

Rolling forward is a little more difficult, but it begins the same way with your knees tucked up and your elbows bent. This time tuck your head forward but raise your hips up over your body from behind. As you do this, you will roll forward to the inverted hang and your shoulders will rotate under your raised hips.

Spotters may assist in a similar manner, but you must tuck your head before they can put their hands on your back.

ROUTINE #1

You are now ready to put these skills together into a simple routine. Start with the rings at eye level and from a side stand under the rings.

1. Jump to a support.
2. Tuck knees and roll forward to a tuck inverted hang.
3. Lower your legs clockwise, stand and inlocate to another tuck inverted hang.
4. Lower your legs again clockwise, and jump to another support.
5. Raise your legs forward with straight knees and hold for three seconds (support L).
6. Roll backwards to a pike inverted hang.
7. Dislocate to stand.
8. Pull your legs up and over your head counterclockwise to a "skin the cat" position.
9. Drop off to a side stand under the rings.

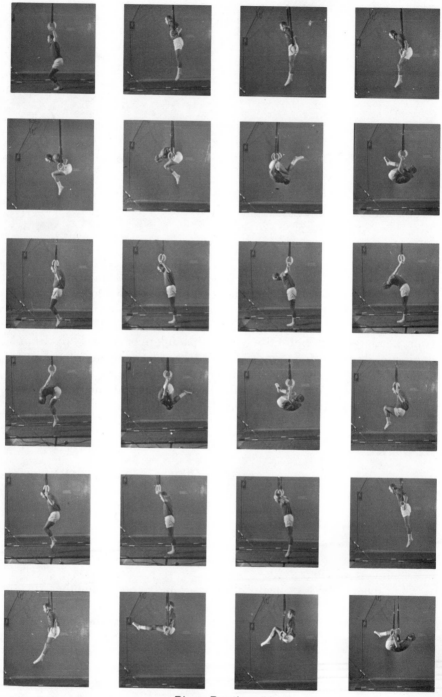

Rings Routine #1.

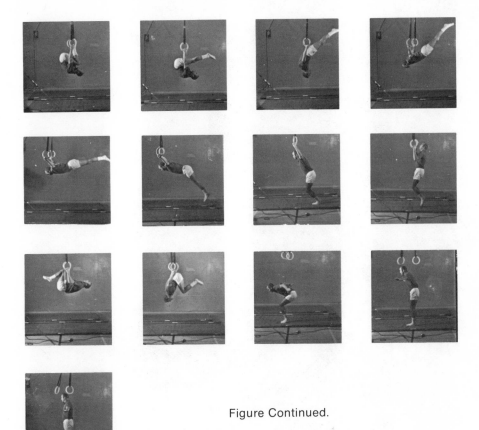

Figure Continued.

KIP

As you have previously learned, the kip can be performed in many of the various events. On the rings, the action is the same (vigorous rapid extension of the hip joint), but it is more difficult because you have no swing to help you gain momentum as on the horizontal bar, and you must hold the rings steady as you perform the skill. It begins from a pike inverted hang and ends in a straight arm support, and may be performed with a normal grip. However, it may be helpful for you to use what is termed a "false grip." In the false grip, the ring goes diagonally across your palm rather than straight across as in the normal grip, and you are supported on the heel of your hand rather than on the middle of your palm. This grip is advantageous because it shortens the length of the lever arm from your shoulder joint to your point of support (heel of hand) and gives you a slight force advantage over the

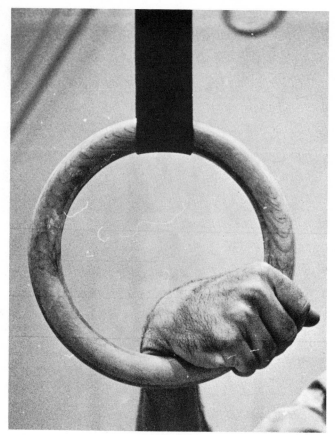

The False Grip.

normal grip. It should be used only for the kip and not for any other skill described in this book, since all other skills are more easily performed with a normal grip.

With a false grip in the pike inverted hang, extend your hips hard and kick your legs forward at about a 45 degree angle from the horizontal. At the same time, roll your head forward and push down on the rings until you come to a bent arm support. Then push up to a straight arm support.

As you gain proficiency, you may kip directly to a straight arm support. Later you may learn this skill with a normal grip. This is one of the more difficult beginning skills on the rings, and can be mastered only after a great deal of practice. Spotters may help you gain the feel of the kip by lifting your upper and lower back as you kick.

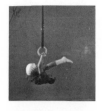
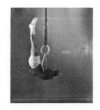
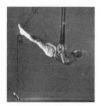
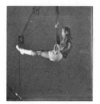

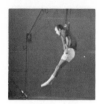
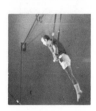

Ring Kip.

ROUTINE #2

The rings should be low when performing this routine. The bottom of the rings should be about even with the top of your head. This routine is the same as Routine #1, except that the kip is substituted for the original jump to support.

1. From a side stand under the rings, pull to a pike inverted hang.
2. Kip to support and. . .
3. Roll forward to a tuck inverted hang.
4. Lower your legs clockwise, and stand and inlocate to another tuck inverted hang.
5. Lower your legs again clockwise and jump to a support.
6. Raise your legs forward with straight knees and hold for three seconds (support L).
7. Roll backwards to a pike inverted hang.
8. Dislocate to stand.
9. Pull your legs up and over your head counterclockwise to a "skin the cat" position.
10. Drop off to a side stand under the rings.

DISLOCATE ON HIGH RINGS

After you have perfected Routine #2, you are ready to learn some skills with the rings placed high enough to enable your body to hang straight without touching the mats.

The dislocate on high rings is performed in the same way as on low rings. You must have mastered the proper technique of shooting your feet up and back while bringing your arms around to the sides

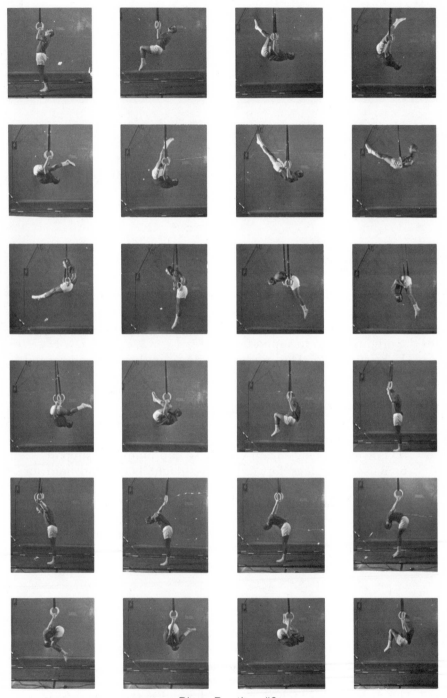

Rings Routine #2.

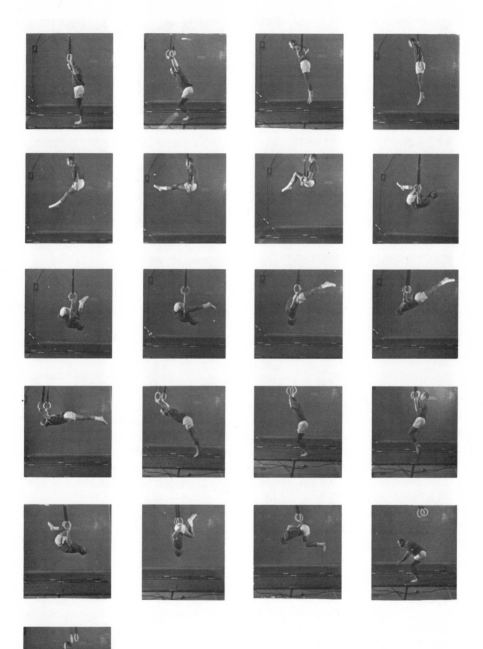

Figure Continued.

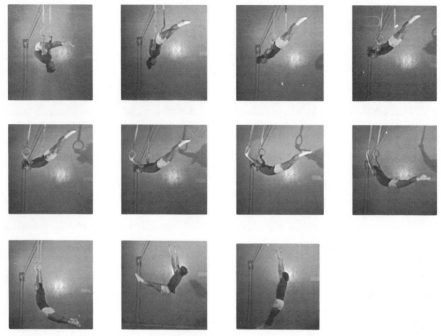

Dislocate on High Rings.

before attempting the dislocate on the high rings. Begin from the pike inverted hand position and extend vigorously, making sure that your arms go out to the sides and then in front of your body. As your legs come down to the hanging position, you may bend your arms slightly to soften the swing when you are first learning, but later on, you should keep your arms straight. The softness of the swing should be accomplished by keeping all of the slack out of the ring straps and keeping your body extended on the underswing.

Spotters can be of great assistance on this move by lifting your shoulders as you extend, and slowing your swing down by lifting up on your thighs.

REAR SWING RISE

This move is performed with a large underswing. As your body swings up in the rear, let your heels rise as high as possible. When they are at their highest point, pull the rings into your body and push up to a support position. In the beginning, you will probably use a great amount of strength to perform this move, but it should really be accomplished with momentum and a minimum amount of strength. The larger the swing, the easier it will be to attain the support position.

(*Text continued on page 116.*)

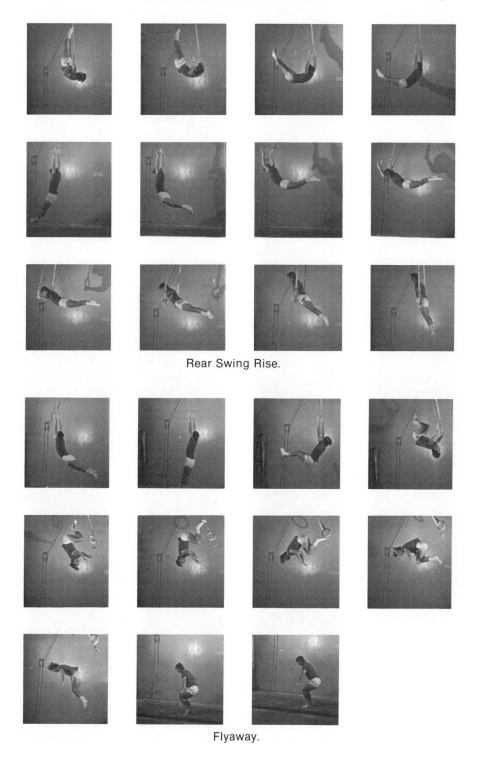

Rear Swing Rise.

Flyaway.

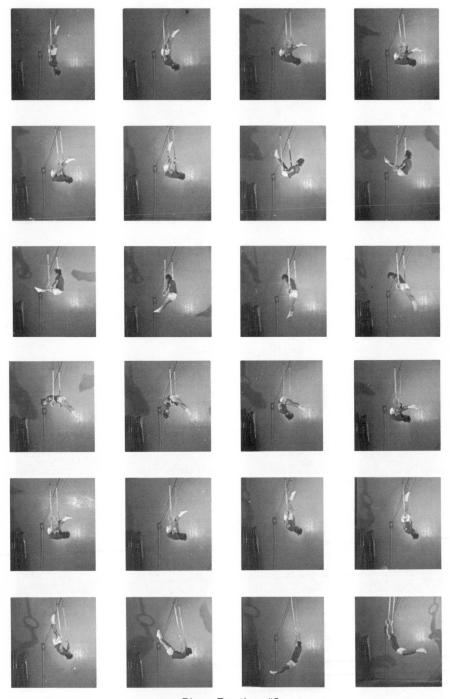

Rings Routine #3.

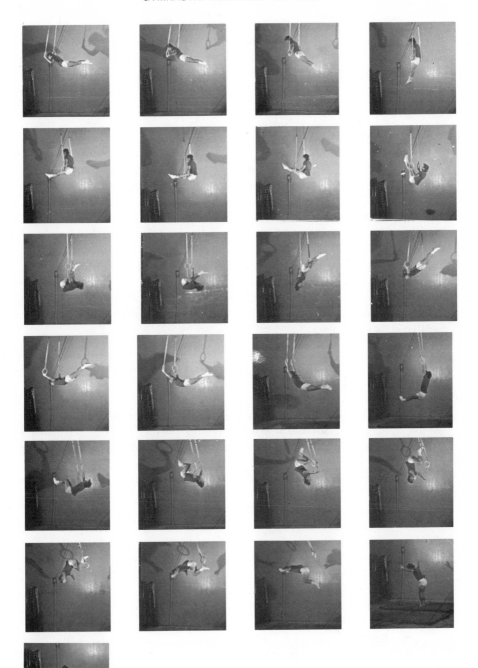

Figure Continued.

After learning it from an underswing, begin in a straight body inverted hang and let your body drop counterclockwise to develop the swing. When doing this, keep your body and arms straight and force the rings backwards or behind your head as your body rotates down.

FLYAWAY

This maneuver on the high rings is nothing more than a swinging "skin the cat," letting go of the rings as your legs pass over your head to start their downward motion. From an underswing, tuck your knees and tilt your head backward on one of the forward swings and look for the mat below. When you see the mat, let go of the rings and complete the somersault in a standing position. When learning, do not let go until you see the mat, but later on you may let go as your feet pass over your head.

Spotters may assist by holding your upper body at the chest and back as you prepare for the landing, or an overhead belt may be utilized.

ROUTINE #3

This may be one of the most difficult routines described in this book, and only with hard work will you perfect it. It is performed with the rings placed high enough for your body to swing under them.

1. From a side stand under the rings, jump to a hang and raise your legs over your head to a pike inverted hang.
2. Kip to a support.
3. Tuck your knees and roll forward to a straight body inverted hang.
4. Lower your body clockwise and swing your legs up in the rear to a. . .
5. Rear swing rise to support.
6. Raise your legs forward to a support L (hold for 3 seconds).
7. Roll backwards (counterclockwise) to a pike inverted hang.
8. Dislocate.
9. Flyaway to a side stand under the rings.

Study the pictures and notice how smoothly one move flows into the next, and how stable and without swing the rings are. If you can perform this routine with ease and agility and "make it look easy," you have certainly met the objectives of the intermediate ring performer.

CHAPTER 9

EVALUATING
PERFORMANCE

Evaluating gymnastics performance in a fair and objective manner is probably one of the most difficult officiating assignments in sports. In competitive gymnastics, the official must not only be knowledgeable about the many different skills that can and are performed on the various pieces of apparatus, but he must be able to identify and classify them according to *difficulty* as they happen. In addition, he must observe the manner in which they are performed and evaluate, in the form of point deductions, each error in *execution* from such minor infractions as failing to keep good posture, to a complete fall from the apparatus. Finally, the judge must concern himself with whether or not the performer met the requirements of the apparatus on which he was working. Failure to perform the required number of handstands, stopping too many times, or leaving out certain specified moves in the event in question results in point deductions for incorrect *combination.*

After considering all of the mechanical aspects of the performance listed above, the judge must then evaluate the total performance on an aesthetic scale to determine whether the gymnast had grace, fluency, style, and poise. In other words, the performer should "make it look easy." All of these things, of course, must be observed, evaluated, and converted into a number score within a few seconds after the gymnast has completed his routine. It is indeed a formidable task, requiring much study and experience.

It is not the purpose of this chapter to train you in this complicated task. For a complete description of the rules and techniques for judging gymnastics, you should refer to the *International Gymnastics Federation (F.I.G.) Code of Points,* distributed by the United States Gymnastics Federation, P.O. Box 4699, Tucson, Arizona. This book represents the most extensive and authoritative source of information available on the subject of judging. In this chapter, a simplified set of rules will be offered to help you evaluate both your own and your classmates' performance on simple optional routines and on the routines listed in this book.

Since the routines described in the previous chapters are structured and set, the difficulty and combination parts of the score will be identical for all who perform them. In a class situation where all are performing one of the routines suggested in this book, the judge need only concern himself with whether or not the routine was performed as written and with the quality, or execution, with which it was performed. This simplifies the judge's task considerably and you should practice in this manner until you are able to give valid and reliable scores on these compulsory routines.

EVALUATING EXECUTION

In order to improve the reliability and validity of the scores the following description of typical execution faults is presented. These descriptions are modified from the *F.I.G. Code of Points,* and are simplified so that you can remember and apply them. You should memorize each of the descriptions and the values of the deductions so that you can write them down from memory as they happen.

Description of Fault	Deduction
1. General poor body position or improper position of hands, arms, legs, feet, or head. (This means poor posture, failure to point toes, spreading of the legs, awkward arm or hand movements, etc.)	.1 to .3
2. Touching the apparatus, uprights, ring straps, mats, etc. with any part of the body when not intended.	.2 to .5
3. Stops, hesitations, or extra swings where not intended.	.2 to .5
4. Sitting, falling, or lying on the apparatus when not intended.	.5 to .7
5. Failure to "make it look easy," such as using too much strength, not enough swing, or too much swing.	.1 to .3
6. Failure to hold intended stops and still positions for 3 seconds. (If a hold is excessively long—over 5 seconds—a deduction may also be made.) .2 for 1 sec. hold, .1 for 2 sec. hold.	.1 to .2

7. Lack of proper technical execution for a skill. (For example, low uprises or kips, lack of sufficient flexibility, lack of rhythm, too many running steps in floor exercise, and anything not mentioned which detracts from the aesthetic value of the performance.)   .1 to .3

8. Failure to dismount with good body control.
   a. One or several steps on landing (.1 per step up to three steps)   .1 to .3
   b. Poor body position even if no steps are taken (bending over too much, excessive waving of arms to maintain balance, etc.).   .1 to .3
   c. Sitting, falling, or kneeling on landing.   .3 to .5

9. Omitting a required move or forgetting a compulsory routine.   .5 to 1.0

10. Falling completely off the apparatus   1.0

Assuming that the maximum value of the routine is ten points, you should write each deduction on a piece of paper as the errors occur, then add them up and subtract from ten to compute the final score.

Each of the deductions refers to a specific move, not to the entire routine. Consequently, the same deductions may be made several times during the routine if the performer commits the same error more than once. Also, notice that each fault has a range of point values from which the judge may select. This is built into the system so that each judge can decide for himself the severity of the fault. For example, if the judge sees what he considers to be a mild failure to point toes, he may deduct only one tenth, but if the performer completely flexes his ankles, and "hooks" his toes, the full three tenths may be deducted. Another judge may consider the same error to be only a two tenths deduction. Hence, the judges are free to interpret the magnitude of the fault and deduct accordingly. This may result in some variation in the judges' scores, but after a little experience, most judges will be able to be quite consistent in their scores and probably will not vary more than five tenths from each other on their final score.

When the performers are executing optional routines with different moves, each of varying difficulty, this flexibility in the deductions allows for a minimal deduction if the move where the fault occurred is a very difficult one. If the same error is committed on an easy move, the judge may elect to impose the maximum deduction.

EVALUATING DIFFICULTY

If the students in your class wish to vary the suggested routines, or to make up their own optional routine (and this is highly recommended when your level of skill becomes sufficient for this to occur), then some provision in the judging must be made to account for the differences in difficulty of the optional routines. In this case, it is suggested that all of the skills that may be used be classified into one of three categories of difficulty: A for easy moves, B for intermediate difficulty moves, and C for maximum difficulty moves. This classification may be suggested by your teacher, or it can be developed by the class. Once it is established, the various moves can be given a point value and a criterion for difficulty may be set. For example, to receive full value for difficulty, you may decide that a routine must contain six A moves, four B moves, and at least one C move. If the A's are worth two tenths of a point, the B's are worth four tenths of a point, and the C's are worth six tenths of a point, then a routine with only five A's and four B's has a maximum value of 9.2 (10.0 minus .6 for the missing C and .2 for the missing A). For this routine, deductions for execution faults would start from 9.2 instead of 10.0.

In this manner, any routine can be analyzed for its component A's, B's, and C's and its ultimate value determined. Of course, more difficult moves may be substituted for easier moves (two C's, three B's and six A's would be acceptable), but as a general rule, easy moves should not substitute for more difficult ones. If a performer has numerous extra B's and C's, he does not receive extra difficulty points, but the deductions for execution faults would be of the minimal amount. Extra difficulty is not usually recommended, because it tends to make the performer try moves that may be beyond his capacity to perform well; hence, he may lose points on the rule that he "fails to make it look easy." Correct execution should never be sacrificed for an increase in difficulty. See if you can answer the following question: What is the maximum value of a routine that contains at least six A's but no B's and C's? (Answer 7.8: 10.0 minus .6 for the missing C and 1.6 for the four missing B's.)

This type of evaluation of difficulty is used in competitive gymnastics and is explained in the *F.I.G. Code of Points*, but the difficulty ratings of the moves are considerably higher than they would be for your class. This is why you must determine your own difficulty ratings, and make them comensurate with the level of ability in your class. Of course, if you are all performing the same routine, difficulty may be ignored and the entire score based on execution alone.

SELECTION OF THE JURY OF JUDGES

Since one of the objectives of a good gymnastics class is to develop appreciation of the sport from a spectator point of view, all members of the class should practice and become proficient at judging. This can be accomplished by letting them practice judging each other during class time and actually serving as the evaluators of the routines when testing and grading is required. Assuming all have had sufficient practice and instruction to judge effectively, the teacher should place the whole class in front of the testing apparatus and select seven students at random to be the judges. Each should be given a judge's score card with numbers ranging from 0 to 10.0 by tenths of a point. When the performance is complete, each judge computes his score, finds it on his score card, and holds it in the air for all to see. A secretary then records all seven scores, eliminates the highest and lowest scores and adds the middle five. The total for the middle five is the contestant's score, and is used to grade the student on that event. The teacher may add his own score to the total or arrange some way for his evaluation to count. By using this method of grading, the students are learning to judge, and are serving as their own peer evaluators. A second attempt at the routine may be offered, with the highest of the two scores to count. Seven different judges should be selected for this second trial.

The author has tried this technique, and has found that the students can become very proficient judges with the final total of five scores being quite valid and reliable. In addition, it stimulates the interest of the class to observe and enjoy gymnastics as a spectator. Such a graduate from a beginning or intermediate gymnastics class benefits not only himself, but the sport of gymnastics as well.

CHAPTER 10

TERMINOLOGY

Axis
An imaginary straight line passing through the body around which the body may revolve. The breadth axis passes from side to side, the depth axis from front to back, and the length axis from head to foot.

Backward
In a counterclockwise direction (see chapter 1).

Balance
A position of static or dynamic support wherein the center of gravity of the body is above the point of support.

Belt
A mechanical device tied around the waist of the performer, usually with ropes attached to the sides so that a spotter can support the performer during gymnastics maneuvers. A twisting belt allows the performer to rotate around the breadth and length axes of his body simultaneously.

Cast
A movement in which the center of gravity of the body is propelled forward or backward to a high position where gravity is allowed to pull it down again for the purpose of developing momentum for some subsequent move.

Center of gravity
That point of the body around which the weight of the body appears to act. In a straight body position it is located at approximately the center of the pelvis. In other positions it may lie outside the body.

Chalk
Carbonate of magnesia, which when placed on the hands absorbs perspiration and thus increases the coefficient of friction between the hands and the apparatus being grasped.

Circle
Rotation or circumduction of one or both arms or legs around some apparatus.

Croup
That part of the side horse between the right end and the right pommel as the gymnast stands facing the horse ready to mount.

Cut
Passing one or both legs under one or both arms with the concomitant weight shift.

False grip
A grip on the rings in which the point of contact between the ring and the hand is nearer the wrist than the center of the palm. This shortens the lever arm between the shoulder joint and the contact point and allows the performer to exert more force.

Feint
A movement on the side horse or horizontal bar in which one or both legs are swung in one direction, and then quickly returned in the opposite direction to develop momentum. These moves are usually detrimental to a good performance and are used mostly as helps in early learning.

Flexibility	The ability of a joint to move. Good flexibility requires the joint to move through its full natural range of motion.
Forward	In a clockwise direction (see chapter 1).
Hang	A position of static or dynamic support wherein the center of gravity of the body is below the point of support.
Judge	An expert who evaluates the performance of a gymnast and converts the results into a numerical score.
Kip	A vigorous, rapid extension of the hip joint designed to create momentum for raising the center of gravity of the body. Kips may be performed forward (clockwise) or backward (counterclockwise) with either the legs or the upper body as the moving part and the other as the stabilizing part.
Lay out	A straight body position.
Momentum	Mass times velocity. Since the mass of the body is relatively constant, increases in momentum are almost always the result of increases in velocity of certain body parts or of the whole body.
Neck	That part of the side horse between the left end and the left pommel as the gymnast stands facing the horse ready to mount.
Pike	A position of the body in which the hip joint is flexed, but the knee joint is straight.
Pommel	The handles of the side horse. With the pommels removed, the side horse becomes a vaulting horse.
Rebound tumbling	Another name for performing tumbling maneuvers on the trampoline.
Roll	A traveling rotation around the breadth or length axis of the body with continual support from the floor or some apparatus.
Saddle	That part of the side horse located between the pommels.
Scissor	A cut of both legs simultaneously (usually on the side horse) with one moving forward and one moving backward.
Somersault	Rotation of 360° or more around the breadth or depth axis of the body.
Spot	The manipulation of a performer either by direct use of the spotter's hands, or by means of a belt placed around the waist of the performer.
Strength	The ability of a muscle or muscles to exert force against resistance.
Swing rise	A maneuver using the swing of the body to develop momentum for the purpose of raising the center of gravity.
Tuck	A position of the body in which the hip and knee joints are flexed. Sometimes the hands grasp the shins.
Twist	Rotation around the length axis of the body.

BIBLIOGRAPHY

BOOKS

Baley, James A., *Gymnastics in the Schools,* Allyn and Bacon, Boston, 1965, 297 pp.
Hughes, Eric, *Gymnastics for Men,* Ronald Press, New York, 1966, 477 pp.
Loken, Newton, and Willoughby, Robert J., *Complete Book of Gymnastics,* Prentice
  Hall, Englewood Cliffs, N.J., 1959, 212 pp.
Maddux, Gordon, *Men's Gymnastics,* Goodyear, Pacific Palisades, Calif., 1970, 82 pp.

PERIODICAL

The Modern Gymnast Magazine, Sunby Publications, 410 Broadway, Santa Monica,
  Calif. 90401.

FILMS

The following 12 minute, color, instructional films are available from Associated
Film Studios, 3419 W. Magnolia Blvd., Burbank, Calif.
  Tumbling and Floor Exercise
  Parallel Bars, Beginning Exercises
  Side Horse, Beginning Exercises
  Horizontal Bar, Beginning Exercises
  Rings, Beginning Exercises
  Trampoline, Beginning Exercises

RULE BOOK

International Gymnastics Federation (F.I.G.) *Code of Points.*
  This rule book is available from the United States Gymnastics Federation, Box
  4699, Tucson, Arizona.